Recent Advances in

Surgery
31

Edited by

Colin D. Johnson MChir FRCS

Reader and Consultant Surgeon, University Surgical Unit, Southampton
General Hospital, Southampton, UK

Irving Taylor MD ChM FRCS FMedSci FRCPS(Glas) FHEA

Vice-Dean and Director of Clinical Studies
Professor of Surgery, Royal Free and University College London Medical
School, University College London, London, UK

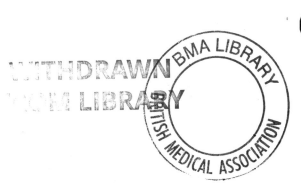
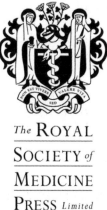

The ROYAL
SOCIETY *of*
MEDICINE
PRESS *Limited*

© 2008 Royal Society of Medicine Press Ltd

Published by the Royal Society of Medicine Press Ltd
1 Wimpole Street, London W1G 0AE, UK
Tel: +44 (0)20 7290 2921
Fax: +44 (0)20 7290 2929
Email: publishing@rsm.ac.uk
Website: www.rsmpress.co.uk

British Library Cataloguing in Publication Data
A catalogue record for this book is available from the British Library
ISBN 978–1–85315–719–6

Distribution in Europe and Rest of World:

Marston Book Services Ltd
PO Box 269, Abingdon
Oxon OX14 4YN, UK
Tel: +44 (0)1235 465500
Fax: +44 (0)1235 465555
Email: direct.order@marston.co.uk

Distribution in the USA and Canada:

Royal Society of Medicine Press Ltd
c/o BookMasters Inc
30 Amberwood Parkway
Ashland, OH 44805, USA
Tel: +1 800 247 6553/+1 800 266 5564
Fax: +1 419 281 6883
Email: order@bookmasters.com

Distribution in Australia and New Zealand:

Elsevier Australia
30-52 Smidmore Street
Marrickville NSW 2204, Australia
Tel: +61 2 9517 8999
Fax: +61 2 9517 2249
Email: service@elsevier.com.au

Editorial services and typesetting by GM & BA Haddock, Ford, Midlothian, UK

Printed in Great Britain by Bell & Bain, Glasgow, UK

Recent Advances in

Surgery
31

Recent Advances in Surgery 30
Edited by I. Taylor & C. D. Johnson

ISBN 978-1-85315-720-2

Contents

Contributors

Sayed Aly PhD FRCS
Consultant Vascular and Endovascular Surgeon, Beaumont/Mater University Hospital, Dublin, Eire

Gary K. Atkin MRCS MD
Specialist Registrar, General Surgery, North-West Thames Region, UK

Stephen Barker MS FRCS
Senior Lecturer in Surgery and Consultant Vascular Surgeon, University College London, London, UK

Andrew R. Bateman MRCP FRCR PhD
Senior Lecturer/Honorary Consultant Clinical Oncologist, University of Southampton, Somers Cancers Sciences Building, Southampton General Hospital, Southampton, UK

Nicholas E. Beck PhD FRCS
Consultant Colorectal Surgeon, Department of Surgery, Southampton General Hospital, Southampton, UK

Emily Boyle MRCS
Research Fellow, National Surgical Training Centre, Royal College of Surgeons in Ireland, Dublin, Eire

Tim J.C. Bryant BMedSci MRCP FRCR
Fellow in Interventional Radiology, Department of Radiology, Southampton General Hospital, Southampton, UK

John A.C. Buckels CBE MD FRCS
Professor of Hepatobiliary and Transplant Surgery, Liver Unit, Queen Elizabeth Hospital, Edgbaston, Birmingham, UK

James A. Catton MD FRCS
Specialist Registrar, Division of Gastrointestinal Surgery, Wolfson Digestive Diseases Centre, Nottingham University Hospitals, Queen's Medical Centre, Nottingham, UK

Udi Chetty BSc MB ChB FRCS MRCP
Consultant Surgeon, Edinburgh Breast Unit, Western General Hospital, Edinburgh, UK

Rowan J. Collinson FRACS
Clinical Colorectal Research Fellow, Department of Colorectal Surgery, The John Radcliffe Hospital, Oxford, UK

Miguel A. Cuesta MD
Professor of Gastro-intestinal Surgery, Department of Surgery, Academic Hospital Vrije Universiteit, Amsterdam, The Netherlands

Hassan Elberm MRCS
Clinical Fellow in HPB surgery, University Surgical Unit, Southampton General Hospital, Southampton, UK

Anthony G. Gallagher BSc PhD
Professor of Human Factors, National Surgical Training Centre, The Royal College of Surgeons in Ireland, Dublin, Eire

Mohammad Abu Hilal MD
Consultant Hepatobiliary Pancreatic and Laparoscopic Surgeon, Honorary Senior Lecturer, School of Medicine, Southampton University Hospital, Southampton, UK

Samer Humadi FRCS
Specialist Registrar, Department of Upper Gastrointestinal and Bariatric Surgery, Musgrove Park Hospital, Taunton, Somerset, UK

Colin D. Johnson MChir FRCS
Reader in Surgery and Consultant Surgeon, University Surgical Unit, Southampton General Hospital, Southampton, UK

Dileep N. Lobo MS DM FRCS
Associate Professor and Reader, Division of Gastrointestinal Surgery, Wolfson Digestive Diseases Centre, Nottingham University Hospitals, Queen's Medical Centre, Nottingham, UK

Jeremy I. Livingstone FRCS MS
Consultant Surgeon, Department of Upper Gastrointestinal Surgery, Watford General Hospital, Watford, Hertfordshire, UK

Fiona McCaig BSc(Hons) MBChB
Research Fellow, Edinburgh Breast Unit, Western General Hospital, Edinburgh, UK

John McHale MD FAA
Consultant Neuro-anaesthethist, Mater University Hospital, Dublin, Eire

Neil J. McC. Mortensen MD FRCS
Professor of Colorectal Surgery, The John Radcliffe Hospital, Oxford, UK

Alistair F. Myers MSc MRCS
Specialist Registrar in Colorectal Surgery, Department of Surgery, Southampton General Hospital, Southampton, UK

Gabriel C. Oniscu MD FRCS
Specialist Registrar, Liver Unit, Queen Elizabeth Hospital, Edgbaston, Birmingham, UK

Daniel O'Leary BSc FRCS FRCS(Gen)
Consultant Colorectal Surgeon, Queen Alexandra Hospital, Portsmouth, UK

Sangeeta A. Paisey MBBS MRCP(UK)
Specialist Registrar Clinical Oncology, Cancer Care Directorate, Southampton General Hospital, Southampton, UK

Amjad Parvaiz FRCS FRCS(Gen Surg) (for correspondence)
Consultant Colorectal Surgeon, Centre for Training in Laparoscopic Colorectal Surgery, Queen Alexandra Hospital, Portsmouth, UK

Lashan Peiris MRCS
Surgical Registrar, Southampton University Hospital, Southampton, UK

Tahseen Qureshi FRCS FRCS(Gen Surg)
Fellow Laparoscopic Colorectal Surgery, Queen Alexandra Hospital, Portsmouth, UK

Roberto Salvia MD PhD
Consultant Pancreatic Surgeon, Verona University Hospital, Verona, Italy

Marcello Spampinato MD
Senior Clinical Fellow in HPB surgery, University Surgical Unit, Southampton General Hospital, Southampton, UK

Irving Taylor MD ChM FMedSci FRCPS(Glas) FHEA
Vice-Dean and Director of Clinical Studies, Professor of Surgery, Royal Free and University College Medical School, London, UK

Richard Welbourn MD FRCS
Consultant Gastrointestinal Surgeon, Department of Upper Gastrointestinal and Bariatric Surgery, Musgrove Park Hospital, Taunton, Somerset, UK

Donald van der Peet MD PhD
Department of Surgery, Academic Hospital Vrije Universiteit, Amsterdam, The Netherlands

Alexander A.F.A. Veenhof MD
Department of Surgery, Academic Hospital Vrije Universiteit, Amsterdam, The Netherlands

Anthony G. Gallagher Emily Boyle

1

Virtual reality simulation in surgery for objective assessment, education, and training

Computer-based simulation has been used for decades in aviation and other professional fields. However, the last 15 years have seen numerous attempts to introduce computer-based simulation into clinical medicine. Surgery, and specifically minimally invasive surgery, has led the way in the development and application of this technology in clinical practice . This style of operating lends itself to virtual reality simulation as the surgeon looks at a video image and not directly at the patient. A simulator can thus be easily created by replacing the video image with a computer model. Recently, use of computer-based simulation for training has expanded into the multidisciplinary fields of catheter-based, image-guided intervention, enabling both surgeons and non-surgeons alike to train on new procedures.

Key point 1

- The traditional Halstedian training model is no longer adequate for training the image-guided interventional skills that are required in laparoscopic surgery.

The first virtual reality surgical simulator in laparoscopic surgery was designed by Satava (Fig. 1).[1] He developed it primarily as a training tool to help counteract the difficulties he observed many of his colleagues were

Anthony G. Gallagher BSc PhD (for correspondence)
Professor of Human Factors, National Surgical Training Centre, The Royal College of Surgeons in Ireland, 123 St Stephen's Green, Dublin 2, Eire
E-mail: aggallagher@rcsi.ie

Emily Boyle MRCS
Research Fellow, National Surgical Training Centre, The Royal College of Surgeons in Ireland, 123 St Stephen's Green, Dublin 2, Eire.

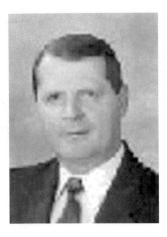 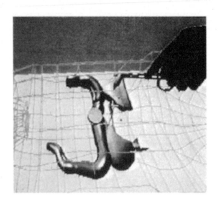

Fig. 1 The first virtual reality simulator created and funded by Prof. Richard Satava in 1991 during his first stint at DARPA.

having in acquiring the skills for laparoscopic surgery. These difficulties were both human-factor and ergonomic in nature, and included issues such as loss of three-dimensional vision, decreased haptic feedback, scaling difficulties and the fulcrum effect.[2] Traditional, Halstedian training models simply did not train the surgeon adequately in this new skill set. Other issues outside the arena of surgery also focused attention on surgical training; the Kennedy report in the UK[3] and the 'To Err is Human' report[4] in the US brought the issue of medical errors to the public consciousness and reported that better training and the use of objective assessment would be crucial in the reduction of medical errors.

WHAT MAKES A GOOD SIMULATOR?

Initial simulators were limited by technological constraints with virtual graphics which were cartoon-like in appearance. However, there have been numerous developments in virtual reality simulators since 1991, many of which have been reviewed elsewhere.[5] Experience has taught us that most surgeons are very naive when evaluating the functionality of simulators. Surgeons tend to evaluate simulators on a very superficial level, *i.e.* does it look like 'real surgery', rather than how the instruments or tissue behave, how appropriate the metrics are, or, most importantly, how appropriate is the simulation curriculum. In the past, surgeons believed that there were two important requisites of any surgical simulator: (i) an accurate depiction of detail; and (ii) a high level of interactivity. Many felt that organs must be anatomically correct and have appropriate natural properties when grasped, clamped or cut, and that grasping an object without weight, shape or texture made training in a virtual environment insubstantial. However, the best validated virtual reality simulator in medicine, the Minimally Invasive Surgical Trainer in Virtual Reality (MIST VR), has demonstrated these beliefs to be, at least partly, incorrect. The first important lesson to be learned about simulation is that it should be developed by a collaborative group including an

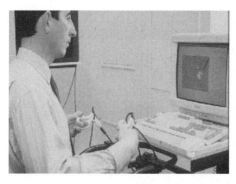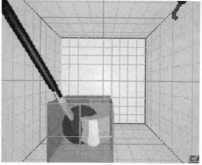

Fig. 2 MIST VR was the first simulator used to demonstrate that proficiency-based virtual reality training improved intra-operative performance in 2002.

engineer, the end-user, (*i.e.* a surgeon) and an expert in curriculum/metrics development (*i.e.* a psychologist). Many simulators are developed by an engineer who has 'consulted' an end-user rather than intimately involving them and rarely are a curriculum developer and a metrics expert involved. Much like a scientific experiment, a simulator is much more difficult to fix at the end of development than at the beginning. For optimal development, these groups need to be intimately involved at the outset. The experts must also be cognisant of the cost implications of their suggestions weighed against what they truly add to the simulation. Lastly, in the development of a simulator, surgeons must give very serious consideration to the fidelity (anatomical realism, haptic feedback and metrics) they require for the accruement of clinical benefit. While one of the advantages of training on a high-fidelity, full-procedural simulator may be additional knowledge accrual, this should not be interpreted as a mandate that all types of computer-based simulation must be high-fidelity. In reality, there are many other means of conveying this knowledge-based information that will be equally or more effective with considerably less cost. One of the requirements of successful implementation of a simulator is, in fact, that the cognitive component of technical skills training should be acquired prior to the psychomotor skills training on the simulator.

Another important point to make about fidelity of a simulator is that fidelity goes beyond computer graphics and presentation. Unfortunately, many surgeons place too much emphasis on the pure graphics aspect of the simulator, or that the simulator looks realistic. It is preferable to have a lower fidelity simulator that trains and assesses simple tasks. Once simple tasks are mastered, then more complex, higher resolution simulations can be performed. The MIST VR system for example, was designed to develop and assess minimally invasive surgical skills using advanced computer technology in a format which could be easily operated by both tutor and trainee (Fig. 2). Although a low-fidelity simulator in that the tasks it sets involve grasping and manipulating targets within a three-dimensional cube, each task develops hand–eye co-ordination and is based on an essential technique employed in minimally invasive surgery.[6]

In a high-fidelity simulation, the tissue and instruments should behave as closely as possible to how they do in a patient. A high-fidelity simulator must

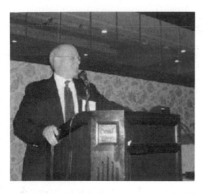 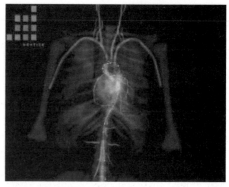

Fig. 3 Dr Steve Dawson and the VIST simulator which started life in his simulation laboratory (CIMIT), MGH and Harvard, in 2007.

allow the trainee to make mistakes (involving both cognitive and psychomotor skills) and learn from these mistakes, and their performance must be meaningfully quantified with well thought out metrics that distinguish between those who are good at the procedure and those who are not. A good example of a high-fidelity simulator in which the model displays similar properties to that of real tissue is the VIST simulator for endovascular procedures such as coronary and carotid stenting (Fig. 3). A robust, but very simple, toolkit of reports for the analysis of performance should be incorporated into the simulator to give clear and easily understood feedback when an error is made. Many simulators available today are hybrid simulators, harnessing augmented reality which is a combination of a real physical model of the patient's viscera and a computer screen showing the virtual operating field (*e.g.* ProMIS™). The surgeon uses real instruments to manipulate the physical model while watching their performance on the screen.

Key point 2

- Surgeons must learn to evaluate simulators and simulation at a more fundamental level than simply asking how 'realistic' it looks. There are more important questions they should ask, such as does it have a curriculum, what metrics are included, how, what and when is feedback given to the trainee? They should also be aware of the price/fidelity elasticity curve.

SIMULATION TRAINING

EVIDENCE-BASED ADOPTION?

Preliminary testing of simulators (such as MIST VR) showed that virtual reality training produced skills that were at least as good as, but usually better than, the conventional training programme.[7] Despite these studies, the surgical community remained unconvinced. Many sceptics pointed to the fact that all of these initial studies simply demonstrated that training on the simulator improved performance on tasks in the skills laboratory and did not demonstrate benefits in operative performance. This was a valid criticism which needed to be addressed. In 2001, a multidisciplinary team at Yale University conducted a prospective, randomised, double-blinded clinical trial to test whether training on a simulator translated into improved intra-operative performance. The trial compared the performance of a group of residents who received standard surgical residency training to a matched group who received proficiency-based training on MIST VR, that is, the residents trained as many trials as necessary to reach the criteria and achieve the qualified proficiency level. Both groups then were objectively assessed on their ability to dissect the gallbladder from the liver bed during a laparoscopic cholecystectomy.[8]

The results of this study showed training on the simulator significantly improved intra-operative performance. Virtual reality trained residents performed the procedure 30% faster and made one-sixth as many objectively assessed intra-operative errors when compared to the standard trained residents. Although the number of subjects was small ($n = 16$), the statistical power of this effect was 0.9996. These results have been independently replicated in Denmark and also in Sweden.[9,10]

The response of the surgical community to the results of this study was mixed; for some, this was enough to convince them that simulation was a powerful training tool. However, the majority clung to the criticism that, while the study was well designed, the small number of subjects, and the fact that only part of the procedure had been performed reduced its wide-spread acceptance. In October 2004 at the Clinical Congress of the American College of Surgeons, another prospective, randomised, double-blinded trial from Emory University was reported that used the same experimental design as the Yale study.[11] However, there were two important differences: (i) in the Emory study, each subject's performance was assessed on the full laparoscopic cholecystectomy procedure; and (ii) the Emory study used only surgical residents in postgraduate years 1 and 2 whereas the Yale study used residents in years 1–4. Again, the virtual reality trained group significantly out-performed the standard trained groups. We believe these results lead to two significant conclusions: (i) simulation, when applied correctly to training, succeeds in improving performance; and (ii) even a low-fidelity virtual reality simulator (such as MIST VR) can produce a very powerful training effect. A similar design was used in the study carried out in Sweden in which residents from postgraduate years 1 and 2 carried out 10 laparoscopic cholecystectomies. The virtual reality-trained group consistently made one-third as many errors and the surgeons in the control group took 58% longer to complete the procedure.[10]

Why does simulation training produce such a powerful training effect? The answers lie in the understanding of the importance of metrics and application of simulation adhering to sound principles of education and training. Further trials are on-going to demonstrate virtual reality to operating room skills transfer on larger groups of subjects and for longer, more complex operative procedures such as laparoscopic colectomy and carotid stenting with embolic protection. These trials will also examine patient outcome as an end-point.

WHY METRIC-BASED SIMULATION?

Computer-based simulation has several advantages when compared with conventional methods for surgical training. One of the major advantages of computer-based simulation is that the same experience or sequence of events can be replicated repeatedly, which allows the trainee to learn from mistakes in a safe environment. Another benefit which is probably equally, if not more, important is the objective feedback a trainee receives from a computer-based simulator. Since everything a trainee 'does' on a computer-based simulator is essentially data, all actions can be tracked by the computer. In addition to crude measures such as performance time, detailed data such as instrument path length, efficiency of instrument movement, and the exact location in space of any instrument at any point in time are recorded. While these data alone are meaningless, they can be used by subject matter experts to create a set of very robust and objective performance metrics. A simulator without metrics is really no better than an expensive video game. While the main function of metrics is to provide the trainee with objective and proximate feedback on their performance, they also allow the trainer to assess objectively the progress of the trainee throughout the training process. This allows the trainer to provide formative feedback to aid the trainee in acquiring a skill. While providing this formative feedback is currently the most valuable function of objective assessment with simulation, inevitably simulators will be used for summative performance assessment. This testing will then be used for processes such as selection and credentialing in the future, much like knowledge testing is used now. In order for simulators to be applied to such high-stakes assessment, it will require a much more rigorous set of metrics. This is still in the experimental phase. When this does come to the fore, it is certain the metrics for that simulator must be shown to meet the same psychometric standards of validation as any other psychometric test.[12]

Some groups[13-15] have been using different metrics (such as performance variability and errors) as a key indicator of skill level. Senior or experienced surgeons perform well, consistently – the reduction of variability is an important aspect of a proficient surgeon, so training to be consistent is as important as training to be proficient. However, the most valuable metric that a simulation can provide is identification of errors. The whole point of training is to improve performance, make performance consistent and reduce errors. Simulation designers must take great care to create error metrics that both train safe behaviour as well as not allowing unsafe behaviour. As simulators permit trainees to commit errors in a consequence-free environment, it is important that dangerous behaviours are not trained. The end result of a good simulator with well-designed metrics is a training system where trainees can learn both what to do and what not to do when operating on patients. In the didactic part of the curriculum, the student must be taught exactly what the error is, and then should be tested to ensure that they are able to identify when they make an error, before starting on the simulator. The errors must be quantified so as to be completely unambiguous. Without robust metrics, the simulator may become a means to train for an adverse outcome waiting to happen.

Key point 4
- Any simulator that does not include appropriate, valid reliable and objective feedback on performance (*i.e.* metrics) is nothing more than an expensive video game.

VIRTUAL REALITY SIMULATION

AN EFFICIENT TOOL FOR DELIVERY OF A PROFICIENCY-BASED CURRICULUM IN SURGERY

Whether a high-fidelity full procedural or low-fidelity basic training simulator is purchased, it should be remembered that it is only a tool which must be integrated into a well-developed curriculum to be effective. Inappropriate application of simulation will lead the user to the erroneous belief that simulation does not work. So how should simulators be appropriately applied to a training curriculum? The goal of current simulation-based training is to create a pre-trained novice.[16] This term describes an individual who may have little, or no, experience with performing the actual procedure, but who has trained to the point where many of the required fundamental skills have already been mastered. With this accomplished, the trainee can devote nearly all of his or her attentional resources to learning the details of performing the actual procedure such as how to identify the correct dissection planes or how to gain exposure in the operative field instead of concentrating on what his or her hands are doing. This results in optimisation of the operating room experience, reduces frustration of both the trainee and mentor, and should result in accelerated learning.

To achieve this goal, a training curriculum must be structured to optimise the skills gained from the simulator. As a guide to curriculum development, the design of any curriculum should contain 6 sequential parts: (i) anatomy instruction; (ii) steps of the procedure; (iii) identification of errors; (iv) a test to insure cognitive knowledge; (v) skills training and assessment on the simulator; and (vi) results reporting and feedback to student.

Key point 5
- Virtual reality simulation is a powerful tool for the delivery of surgical training within a curriculum.

PROFICIENCY-BASED PROGRESSION TRAINING

The traditional way that simulation has been applied to training is through a prescriptive approach. Typically, the trainee is required to train for a pre-specified number of trials or number of hours. However, all that this approach achieves is considerable variability in post-training skills.[16] Individuals start from different baseline skill levels, they learn at different rates and some are more gifted than others. Simulation allows for levelling of the playing field and sets a skill 'benchmark' which individuals can reach at their own pace. They should also not be allowed to progress to the next phase of training until they demonstrate that they are performing proficiently and consistently. Using the carefully developed metrics and setting the criteria by which the proficiency level is determined, the simulator can then objectively assess and quantify the performance of the proficient individual. This objectively determined 'proficiency level' can then be used as a goal for those training on the simulator; in fact, this is the key aspect of implementing a successful simulation training curriculum. Training on the simulator should not be complete until the trainee has reached an objectively established level of proficiency.

When setting the proficiency level, the surgeons used to set the standard need not be the best of the best; rather, they should reflect a representative sample of the proficient population. If the proficiency level is set too high, trainees will never reach it; if set too low, an inferior skills set will be produced. Ideally, proficiency levels would be set nationally or internationally. While national or international proficiency levels on virtual reality simulators may be some way off, proficiency levels can be set locally in each training programme or hospital. The Yale and Emory virtual reality to operating room studies and the Swedish study have all shown the power of this approach.[8–10] The whole point of training is not simply to improve performance but also to make it more consistent. Indeed, performing well consistently is emerging as one of the key indicators of training success.[8,13]

Proficiency-based training as a new approach to the acquisition of procedural-based medical skills took a giant leap forward in April 2004. As part of the roll-out of a new device for carotid angioplasty and stenting, the US Food and Drug Administration (FDA) mandated, as part of the device approval package, metric-based training to proficiency on a virtual reality simulator as the required training approach for physicians who will be using the new device.[17] The company manufacturing the carotid stent system informed the FDA that they would educate physicians with a tiered training approach using an on-line, multimedia, didactic package and training of catheter- and wire-handling skills with a high-fidelity virtual reality simulator using a curriculum based on achieving a level of proficiency in both the didactic and technical areas. What this approach allows is for training of physicians who enter training with variable knowledge, skill, and experience, but leave with objectively assessed proficient knowledge and skills. This is particularly important for a procedure like carotid angioplasty and stenting as it crosses multiple clinical specialties with each bringing a different skill set to the training table. A sound training strategy must ensure that all of these specialists are able to meet an objectively assessable minimum level of proficiency in all facets of the procedure. We believe that this development represents a paradigm shift in the way procedural-based medicine is trained and will result in a reduction in 'turf wars' concerning future credentialing for new procedures. As long as a physician is able to demonstrate that he or she possesses the requisite knowledge and skills to perform a procedure, specialty affiliation will become irrelevant. Overall, we see this development as a good thing for surgery, procedural-based medicine and for patient safety.

Key point 6

- Virtual reality simulation does not work by osmosis. Published evidence clearly indicates that the optimal approach to using this tool is to use objective benchmarking or proficiency levels that are based on the performance of experienced surgeons currently practising this type of surgery.

CONCLUSIONS

Computer-based simulation or virtual reality simulation has been around for more than a decade, but has only recently begun to gain momentum. Despite considerable early scepticism, there is now a growing body of evidence to show that properly applied computer-based simulation training strategies improve performance of surgical trainees. Developing simulators to produce these results is not easy and must be done collaboratively with experts in computer science, engineering, medicine, and behavioural and educational science to produce a robust training tool. A good simulation is about more than graphics and 'prettiness'. Robust metrics must be in place to help trainees learn both what to do and what not to do. Finally, simulation must be incorporated as a component of an overall education and training curriculum designed to produce trainees with consistently reproducible skills. Simulation is a very powerful tool and surgeons should use it (appropriately).

Key points for clinical practice

- The traditional Halstedian training model is no longer adequate for training the image-guided interventional skills that are required in laparoscopic surgery.

- Surgeons must learn to evaluate simulators and simulation at a more fundamental level than simply asking how 'realistic' it looks. There are more important questions they should ask, such as does it have a curriculum, what metrics are included, how, what and when is feedback given to the trainee? They should also be aware of the price/fidelity elasticity curve.

- There is a growing body of evidence which clearly demonstrates in prospective, randomised, controlled trials, that proficiency-based virtual reality training on simulators provides superior intra-operative skills when compared to the traditional approach.

(continued)

Key points for clinical practice *(continued)*

- The traditional Halstedian training model is no longer adequate for training the image-guided interventional skills that are required in laparoscopic surgery.

- Surgeons must learn to evaluate simulators and simulation at a more fundamental level than simply asking how 'realistic' it looks. There are more important questions they should ask, such as does it have a curriculum, what metrics are included, how, what and when is feedback given to the trainee? They should also be aware of the price/fidelity elasticity curve.

- There is a growing body of evidence which clearly demonstrates in prospective, randomised, controlled trials, that proficiency-based virtual reality training on simulators provides superior intra-operative skills when compared to the traditional approach.

- Any simulator that does not include appropriate, valid reliable and objective feedback on performance (*i.e.* metrics) is nothing more than an expensive video game.

- Virtual reality simulation is a powerful tool for the delivery of surgical training within a curriculum.

- Virtual reality simulation does not work by osmosis. Published evidence clearly indicates that the optimal approach to using this tool is to use objective benchmarking or proficiency levels that are based on the performance of experienced surgeons currently practising this type of surgery.

References

1. Satava RM. Virtual reality surgical simulator; the first steps. *Surg Endosc* 1993; **7**: 203–205.
2. Gallagher AG, Smith CD. Human-factors lessons learned from the minimally invasive surgery revolution. *Semin Laparosc Surg* 2003; **10**: 100–110.
3. Senate of Surgery. *Response to the General Medical Council Determination on the Bristol Case.* London: Senate Paper 5, The Senate of Surgery of Great Britain and Ireland, 1998.
4. Kohn LT, Corrigan JM. *To Err is Human: Building a Safer Heath System.* Washington, DC. Institute of Medicine, 1999.
5. Schijven M, Jakimowicz J. Virtual reality surgical laparoscopic simulators. *Surg Endosc* 2003; **12**: 1943–1950.
6. Wilson MS, Middlebrook A, Sutton C, Stone R, McCloy RF. MIST VR: a virtual reality trainer for laparoscopic surgery assesses performance. *Ann R Coll Surg Engl* 1993; **75**: 403–404.
7. Gallagher AG, McClure N, McGuigan J, Crothers I, Browning J. Virtual reality training in laparoscopic surgery; a preliminary assessment of Minimally Invasive Surgical Trainer Virtual Reality (MIST VR). *Endoscopy* 1999; **31**: 310–313.
8. Seymour N, Gallagher AG, Roman S *et al.* Virtual reality training improves operating room performance: results of a randomized, double-blinded study. *Ann Surg* 2002; **236**: 458–464.
9. Grantcharov TP, Kristianson VB, Bendix J, Bardram L, Rosenerg J, Funch-Jensen P. Randomized clinical trial of virtual reality simulation for laparoscopic skills training. *Br J Surg* 2004; **91**: 146–150.

10. Ahlberg G, Enochsson L. Proficiency-based virtual reality training reduces the error rate for residents during their first 10 laparoscopic cholecystectomies. *Am J Surg* 2007; **193**: 797–804.

11. McClusky DA, Gallagher AG, Ritter EM *et al*. Virtual reality training improves junior residents' operating room performance: results of a prospective randomized double-blinded study of the laparoscopic cholecystectomy. *J Am Coll Surg* 2004; **199 (Suppl)**: 73.

12. Gallagher AG, Ritter EM, Satava RM. Fundamental principles of validation, and reliability: rigorous science for the assessment of surgical education and training. *Surg Endosc* 2003; **10**: 1525–1529.

13. Gallagher AG, Satava RM. Objective assessment of experienced, junior and novice laparoscopic performance with virtual reality: learning curves and reliability measures. *Surg Endosc* 2002; **16**: 1746–1752.

14. Ritter E, McClusky D, Gallagher A *et al*. Objective psychomotor skills assessment of experienced and novice flexible endoscopists with a virtual reality simulator. *J Gastrointest Surg* 2003; **7**: 871–878.

15. Tang B, Hanna GB, Joice P, Cuschieri A. Identification and categorization of technical errors by Observational Clinical Human Reliability Assessment (OCHRA) during laparoscopic cholecystectomy. *Arch Surg* 2004; **139**: 1215–1220.

16. Gallagher AG, Ritter EM, Champion H *et al*. Virtual reality simulation for the operating room: proficiency-based training as a paradigm shift in surgical skills training. *Ann Surg* 2005; **24**: 364–372.

17. Gallagher AG, Cates CU. Approval of virtual reality training for carotid stenting: what this means for procedural-based medicine. *JAMA* 2004; **292**: 3024–3026.

James A. Catton Dileep N. Lobo

2

The use of drains in gastrointestinal surgery

The *Oxford English Dictionary* defines a drain as 'a channel by which surplus liquid is drained or gradually carried off'. While this definition can be applied satisfactorily to a surgical drain, nothing can be further from the truth than the second half of the definition offered by the online encyclopaedia, *Wikipedia* in 2007: 'Drains inserted after surgery help the wound to heal faster and assist in preventing infection'. Unfortunately, this misconception is ingrained in the minds of many surgeons.

Most surgeons have strong opinions on the use of drains and the majority develop these opinions based on their own personal experience and those of their predecessors. Robinson[1] aptly classified surgeons into three categories based on their use of drains: those who believe that all intraperitoneal operations should be drained, those who feel that drainage is useless and those who sit on the fence and insert a drain as a safety valve or perhaps as a sop to their consciences.

This review explores some of the practical issues associated with drains in gastrointestinal surgery and examines the evidence base for the use of drains in modern surgical practice.

HOW DO DRAINS WORK?

Poiseuille determined that the laminar flow rate of an incompressible fluid along a tube is proportional to the fourth power of the radius of the tube.

James A. Catton MD FRCS
Specialist Registrar, Division of Gastrointestinal Surgery, Wolfson Digestive Diseases Centre,
Nottingham University Hospitals, Queen's Medical Centre, Nottingham NG7 2UH, UK

Dileep N. Lobo MS DM FRCS (for correspondence)
Associate Professor and Reader, Division of Gastrointestinal Surgery, Wolfson Digestive Diseases
Centre, Nottingham University Hospitals, Queen's Medical Centre, Nottingham NG7 2UH, UK
E-mail: dileep.lobo@nottingham.ac.uk

Poiseuille's law states that the flow rate Q is also dependent upon fluid viscosity η, length of the tube L and the pressure difference between the ends P:

$$Q = \frac{\pi r^4 P}{8 \eta L}$$

Hence, while fluid is being produced continuously: (i) flow is directly proportional to the suction pressure (P) applied to the drain, and to the fourth power of the radius of the drain (r); (ii) flow is inversely proportional to the viscosity of the fluid (η) and the length of the drain (L); and (iii) flow can be increased by 16-fold by doubling the radius (or diameter) of the drain and can be doubled by reducing the length of the drain by one half.

Factors that help fluid flow from body cavities to the exterior through drains include gravity, tissue pressure, capillary action and negative pressure (when applied by suction devices).

SIZE

The size of tube drains is often measured by the Charrière system or the French (F) gauge.[2] The number represented by the French gauge is the circumference of the tube in millimetres. For example, a 10-F tube drain has a circumference of 10 mm and a diameter of 3.18 mm (circumference = π x diameter or 2π x radius). At a practical level, the external diameter of a drain can be estimated by dividing the French gauge by 3. Of course, the inner diameter of the drain is (2 x wall thickness) less than the calculated external diameter.

TYPES OF DRAINS

Drains can be classified in a number of ways.

RATIONALE

Prophylactic drains
A drain placed at the end of an operative procedure to prevent accumulation of fluid is called a prophylactic drain. In some cases, such drains are thought to aid in the detection of fluid accumulation or leakage, e.g. from an anastomotic breakdown. As we shall argue later, there is little or no role for the use of prophylactic drainage in gastrointestinal surgery.

Therapeutic drains
A drain placed to evacuate an existing collection (such as a subphrenic abscess) is known as a therapeutic drain. Therapeutic drains may be placed surgically or under radiological guidance.

MECHANISM

Open drains
Open drains are those that drain freely to the exterior and not into a reservoir. There is a risk of bacteria and other organisms ascending along the drain into

the cavity being drained. Open drains such as a Penrose or corrugated drain can be useful in certain situations. As they tend to be softer than tube drains, they are more comfortable for the patient and are less likely to get blocked.

Closed drains
Closed drains allow fluid to drain externally into a sealed container and offer a number of advantages over open drains. As early as the 1960s,[3,4] it was shown that there is a lower risk of infections with closed drains when compared with open drains. In addition, closed drains protect the patient's skin by keeping fluid away from it, they are easier to care for and help provide an accurate assessment of fluid drainage.

Suction versus non-suction (passive) drains
Closed drainage systems can be divided into suction drains where a negative pressure is applied to facilitate drainage (Fig. 1), or passive drains, where fluid is allowed to drain under capillary action, natural pressure gradients or gravity. Suction has a number of advantages. It allows the drainage of fluid from areas where the movement of fluid is against the natural pressure gradient, such as the pleural space; it also helps appose tissue planes, thereby preventing fluid accumulation, and blockage of the drain by debris is less likely (but not impossible!) as a result of the continuously applied negative pressure. The disadvantage of suction drainage is that the suction force applied can cause tissue erosion and can prevent an established fistula from closing by allowing continuous drainage of fluid.

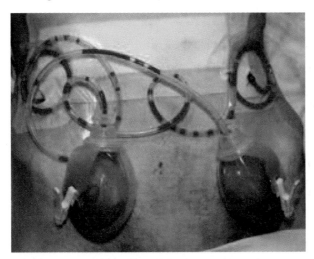

Fig. 1 A closed suction drainage system. There are two drains, each with attached compressible chamber. Evacuation of the chamber by squeezing generates constant, low-pressure suction until the chamber has filled with fluid.

Sump suction versus closed suction
Sump suction involves the use of a double lumen tube, with the second lumen acting as a 'vent' to allow air flow down to the tip of the drain. This prevents negative pressure arising at the tip of the drain and subsequent blockage from

surrounding tissue. This, in turn, reduces the amount of tissue damage. It does, however, result in the system been technically open, with reduced patient mobility due to the need for continuous wall suction.

DRAIN MATERIALS

In the past, drains used to be made of red rubber or latex. These were irritant, and so induced a fibrotic reaction and also had the risk of inducing allergic reactions. Currently, most drains are made of polyurethane, silicone (silastic), silicone elastomer, polytetrafluoroethylene (PTFE) or siliconised latex.[5] Polyurethane is stronger than silicone, allowing for a tube of this material to have thinner walls and thus a larger internal diameter for the same French gauge. The flexibility and decreased internal diameter of silicone tubes may lead to clogging or kinking of the tube. Soft drains are less likely to erode into tissues. A radio-opaque stripe is usually incorporated along the long axis of a drain in order to ensure visibility on X-ray.

WHY USE DRAINS?

In abdominal surgery, drains may be used to provide a route for egress of blood, bile, pus, urine, lymph, pancreatic secretions and bowel contents from anastomotic leaks. Common reasons for using drains are listed in Table 1.

Table 1 Reasons for the insertion of a drain

- To remove unwanted fluid/exudates/pus/gas
- To allow monitoring of fluid volume and quality
- To promote tissue apposition
- To allow diversion of body fluids
- To facilitate subsequent access to a body space or cavity
- To allow the injection of dye or contrast to provide diagnostic information about an underlying cavity or fistula.

Table 2 Things to watch for in a patient with a drain

- Is the patient well?
- Has the drain been secured and is it still secure?
- Are there signs of infection, excoriation or peritubal leakage at the skin exit site?
- Is the tube kinked or damaged?
- Is the drain connected properly?
- What is draining? – volume, colour, nature, smell
- Has there been any change in the nature or volume of the effluent?
  - little or no output indicates that the drain is either blocked or that it has served its function
  - excessive drainage may indicate formation of a fistula or tissue irritation
- Is the vacuum for suction drains working?

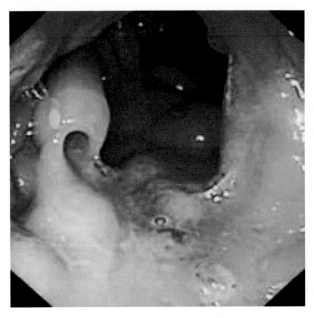

Fig. 2 Leaving a drain *in situ* for too long can lead to complications. This colonoscopic image shows migration of an abdominal drain into the transverse colon.

INSERTION, CARE AND REMOVAL OF DRAINS

All drains should be inserted and removed with care. Drains should be exteriorised by the shortest safe route and should not be brought out through the surgical incision. The size and length of the drain should be appropriate for its purpose and it should be secured firmly at the exit site in order to prevent migration either inwards or outwards. The drain should be inspected daily and particular attention should be paid to the features shown in Table 2.

Drains should never be allowed to outlive their usefulness and the rate of complications increases with the duration of drainage (Fig. 2). Steady gentle traction should be used to remove the drain rather than sudden jerky movements. Suction should be released prior to removal of suction drains.

DRAIN MALFUNCTION

All drains are potentially dangerous and the natural history of a drain is to malfunction.[5] Common complications of abdominal drains are listed in the Table 3. Close monitoring of drains is required at all times to detect problems at their onset. Once a problem is detected, a strategy for tackling the problem should be formulated. Ultimately, the treatment for a malfunctioning drain is almost always its removal!

TO DRAIN OR NOT TO DRAIN? THE EVIDENCE BASE

The use of drains is engrained in surgical practice, but is there evidence in the literature to support their use? For each different area of gastrointestinal surgery, the

Table 3 Common complications of drains

- Tissue damage during insertion and removal
- Erosion into adjacent structures – blood vessels, bowel, anastomoses
- Skin flap necrosis
- Visceral herniation through the drain tract
- Bacterial colonisation and infection
- Loss of fluid and electrolytes (*e.g.* through a T-tube)
- Pain
- Migration or displacement of the drain (into the body cavity or extrusion)
- Accidental removal
- Blockage
- Fracture of the drain
- Failure of vacuum in suction drains
- Restricted patient mobility.

evidence for drain usage is addressed and given a grade of recommendation based on the classification by the Oxford Centre for Evidence-based Medicine.[6]

NASOGASTRIC DRAINAGE

The practice of inserting a nasogastric tube to allow decompression of the gastric contents dates back over 300 years. Its prophylactic use after abdominal surgery is contentious. The arguments offered for routine postoperative use included reduced nausea and vomiting, and reduced abdominal distension leading to a lower risk of aspiration and subsequent pneumonia. There have also been suggestions that abdominal wound complications and infections are also reduced. Nasogastric tubes are notoriously uncomfortable for patients, so is there evidence to support their routine use?

Two meta-analyses looking at the benefits of prophylactic insertion of nasogastric tubes have been have been carried out, the first by Cheatam *et al.*[7] in 1995. This analysis looked at both randomised and non-randomised studies published up to 1995. Other than a slight reduction in the incidence of postoperative nausea and vomiting, no other significant difference in the outcome was evident whether or not a nasogastric tube was placed.[7]

A more up-to-date and rigorous analysis was carried out by Nelson *et al.*[8,9] in 2005 as part of the Cochrane Review process. This study looked at 28 randomised studies that included a total of 4194 patients, of whom 2108 had a nasogastric tube placed routinely. A number of outcomes including return of gastrointestinal function, pulmonary complications, wound infection, ventral hernia and anastomotic leak were looked at. Little difference in outcome was seen with the use of routine nasogastric decompression. The only significant difference was an earlier return of gastrointestinal function, measured by time to passage of flatus and this occurred in those patients in whom a nasogastric tube was not inserted. There was also a suggestion that non-insertion of a nasogastric was associated with fewer respiratory complications but this did not reach statistical significance.

The use of nasogastric tubes should be confined to therapeutic purposes, *e.g.* treatment of acute gastric dilatation, the management of duodenal fistulae, gastric outlet obstruction and small bowel obstruction, and nasogastric feeding.

Key point 1

- The routine use of nasogastric tubes cannot be recommended (Grade A).

COLORECTAL SURGERY

The use of drains in colorectal surgery centres around their effects on colorectal anastomoses. Once an anastomotic leak has occurred, drainage is generally accepted as the treatment of choice. Of greater controversy is the use of prophylactic drainage. The underlying principle of drainage is to prevent fluid accumulation around the anastomosis, thereby preventing infection and subsequent dehiscence. If dehiscence occurs this can be detected early, with an efflux of faeces or purulent fluid from the drain. However, such logic has been questioned by experimental evidence that drainage may in fact lead to greater infection in the anastomotic area.[10]

As part of the Cochrane Review process, Karliczek et al.[11] performed a systematic review and meta-analysis of drainage versus no drainage following colorectal anastomoses. Looking solely at elective surgery, they identified six randomised controlled trials comparing different drainage regimens. A total of 1140 patients were analysed; 573 allocated to drainage and 567 to no drainage. The primary outcome measure was mortality with secondary outcomes of clinical and radiological dehiscence, wound infection, re-intervention and extra-abdominal complications. Mortality was virtually identical – 3% (18 of 573 patients) with drainage, 4% (25 of 567 patients) without. When patients who had drains inserted were compared with those without drains, the rates of radiological anastomotic dehiscence (3% versus 4%), wound infection (5% in both groups), re-intervention (6% versus 5%) and extra-abdominal complications (7% versus 6%) were similar.

The conclusion drawn from this analysis was that the prophylactic drainage was not warranted, although the placement of drains appeared to cause no significant harm. Even with pooling of the data, the study population was small and the main interest group, patients with low colorectal anastomoses, was poorly represented.

Key point 2

- Based on the best available evidence, drainage after routine colorectal surgery cannot be recommended (Grade A).

APPENDICECTOMY

Appendicectomy is one of the commonest gastrointestinal operations performed and, for many, the decision to leave a drain is determined by whether the underlying appendicitis is complicated or not. Drainage following 'simple' appendicitis has been assessed by two randomised trials, the first suggesting an increased incidence of wound infection[12] with the placement of a drain and the second showing no significant difference in any postoperative complications.[13] Both these studies were small and are now relatively historical.

There have been four randomised trials carried out when the appendix was either perforated or gangrenous,[12–15] with a subsequent meta-analysis by Petrowsky *et al.*[16] This showed that both wound infection and the rate of subsequent faecal fistula formation is lower if no drain is left, with the rate of intra-abdominal collection similar in both groups. Again, all the studies included were small and historical; however, they are the best evidence available. No evidence exists as to whether this approach should be extrapolated to laparoscopic appendicectomy.

Key point 3

- The placement of a prophylactic drain following appendicectomy is not indicated, regardless of the severity of appendicitis (Grade A).

CHOLECYSTECTOMY

Data from the era of open cholecystectomy fail to support the use of a prophylactic drain.[13,17–19] A meta-analysis by Lewis *et al.*[20] in 1990 showed no significant reduction in postoperative complications. The recent Cochrane Review goes further and suggests that postoperative drainage not only increases wound infection rates following open cholecystectomy put also increases the incidence of respiratory tract infections.[21] With the onset of laparoscopic cholecystectomy, drain placement studies initially looked at 'gas' drains sited to prevent pain and nausea from redundant gas post-operatively.[22,23] No significant difference in postoperative complications was seen in these studies, and only one showed a small, non-significant reduction in postoperative pain with the placement of a drain.[22] Again, the recent Cochrane Review has strongly recommended avoiding drainage after laparoscopic cholecystectomy citing both increased rates of wound infection and delayed postoperative discharge in patients having uncomplicated operations when drains were placed.[21]

Key point 4

- Prophylactic drain placement cannot be advocated following simple cholecystectomy, either laparoscopic or open (Grade A).

HEPATIC RESECTION

Subphrenic collections and bilomas represent the commonest intra-abdominal complications following liver resection.[24] Prophylactic drainage is the accepted practice following hepatic resection. There have been three randomised controlled trials of prophylactic drainage, all using closed suction drainage systems. Meta-analysis of these trials showed the incidence of postoperative collections was not reduced by the placement of a drain. When a collection does occur, it is more likely to become infected if a drain is present.[16] In addition, the likelihood of percutaneous drain placement postoperatively was not reduced by the initial placement of a prophylactic drain. Drain placement also failed to detect postoperative bile leakage and haemorrhage reliably.[25] The Cochrane Review by Gurusamy et al.,[26] taking in a slightly broader array of trials, has recently confirmed these findings.

Key point 5

- Prophylactic drain placement following liver resection is not beneficial and may even be detrimental (Grade A).

T-TUBE DRAINAGE OF THE COMMON BILE DUCT

T-tube insertion is the traditional management following choledocholithotomy for common bile duct exploration. The rationale for this approach is based on the belief that the T-tube allows decompression of the oedematous common bile duct, preventing biliary leakage. It also allows access for postoperative visualisation and even the retrieval of retained stones.

The evidence to support T-tube placement over primary duct closure is sparse. There are only three randomised controlled trials. All are relatively small and date back to the open era of biliary surgery in the late 1980s and early 1990s. De-Roover et al.[27] randomised only 22 patients to either primary closure or closure over a T-tube and found no difference in outcome between the two groups. Sheen-Chen et al.[28] randomised 30 patients in a similar way and noted that, although most outcome measures were similar, operative time and postoperative stay was longer in the T-tube group. The largest study by Williams et al.[29] from New Zealand included 37 patients undergoing primary closure and 26 having closure over T-tube. Again, outcomes were similar in both groups with those having a T-tube placed having a significantly longer postoperative stay.

Key point 6

- Based on the available evidence, the routine placement of a T-tube following common bile duct exploration cannot be supported (Grade B). However, there may be a case for inserting a subhepatic drain for 24–48 h after closure of the common bile duct.

UPPER GASTROINTESTINAL SURGERY

In benign upper gastrointestinal surgery, there is only a single non-randomised prospective cohort study looking at prophylactic drainage. This was in surgery for perforated duodenal ulcers and included 119 patients: 75 had a drain placed at the discretion of the operating surgeon. There was no difference in the incidence of intra-abdominal collections between the two groups, but there was a 10% incidence of complications associated with drain placement and a 3% rate of intestinal obstruction when a drain was placed.[30]

In upper gastrointestinal oncological surgery, there have been two randomised controlled trials of prophylactic drainage, both from the Far East. One study looked at sub-total and total gastrectomy in 170 patients.[31] There was no difference in 30-day complication rates whether a drain was placed or not. In the second study, 108 patients undergoing subtotal gastrectomy were randomised to routine drainage or not.[32] Again, there was no difference in the postoperative complication rate in either group. Based on these studies, routine drainage following upper gastrointestinal surgery cannot be recommended (Grade B).

PANCREATIC SURGERY

The most frequently performed pancreatic resection is pancreaticoduodenectomy for a lesion in the head of the pancreas. Since Kausch's original description, and Whipple's subsequent modification, prophylactic drainage has a been a standard part of the procedure. This classically involves two drains – one in close proximity to the pancreaticojejunostomy and one by the hepaticojejunostomy. When only the distal pancreas is excised, a drain is traditionally placed near to the resection margin.

There has only been one randomised controlled trial comparing prophylactic drainage with no drainage. This was carried out at the Memorial Sloan-Kettering Hospital by Conlon et al.[33] Patients were randomised to either standard drainage as described above or no drains at all. A total of 179 patients were enrolled with 139 having a pancreaticoduodenectomy and the remainder having a distal pancreatectomy. Not only was the rate of complications lower where no drains were placed but number of interventions for collections was greater when drains had been placed. On the basis of this evidence, the routine placement of drains following pancreatic surgery cannot be recommended (Grade B).

Key point 7

- In upper gastrointestinal and pancreatic surgery there is little evidence to support the use of drains.

DRAIN PLACEMENT AFTER HERNIA REPAIR

Although drain placement is not common after most types of hernia repair, there is some debate over a role following incisional hernia repair. Traditional teaching is that drains have a role in reducing blood and fluid accumulation[34] and that this, in turn, reduces the recurrence of incisional hernias.[35] Some contradict this view claiming no alteration in fluid accumulation rates[36] or incisional hernia rates.[37] There is also a suggestion that drains act as a foreign body and increase the risk of infection.[38] The Cochrane Review carried out by Gurusamy and Samraj[39] failed to clarify the situation. Only a single trial involving drainage following incisional hernia repair could be identified and this compared two types of drains rather than drainage versus no drainage.

Key point 8

- Currently, the placement of drains following incisional hernia repair has to be at the discretion of the operating surgeon.

THERAPEUTIC DRAINAGE

Surgical placement of a therapeutic drain is now rarely performed. This has been principally due to the introduction of percutaneous drainage under image guidance. This most typically takes the form of ultrasound guidance but can also include CT-directed intervention. No trial exists of drainage versus no drainage for postoperative symptomatic collections, as there is consensus that drainage is the only treatment option. The value of percutaneous drainage can, however, be seen with its role in the critically ill patient with acute cholecystitis. Percutaneous cholecystostomy was originally described by Radder[40] in 1980. It has since gone on to form the mainstay of treatment for those patients wiyh unresolving acute cholecystitis unfit to undergo formal cholecystectomy.[41–43]

Key point 9

- Percutaneous drainage is the recommended treatment for symptomatic postoperative collections and when there are signs of infection.

CONCLUSIONS

The role of therapeutic drains is not in doubt. The role of prophylactic drainage is much more uncertain. Despite being an established part of surgical practice, there is little evidence to support the routine use of prophylactic drainage. In all areas of gastrointestinal surgery, evidence exists of Grade B or better that drain placement has no demonstrable benefit. In some cases, drains may even be detrimental.

In practical terms, all drains have a purpose; when that purpose is gone, so should the drain. Drain-related complications are common and are universally treated by removal or replacement of the drain. Maybe the time has come to consider their placement in the first place?

Key points for clinical practice

- The routine use of nasogastric tubes cannot be recommended (Grade A).

- Based on the best available evidence, drainage after routine colorectal surgery cannot be recommended (Grade A).

- The placement of a prophylactic drain following appendicectomy is not indicated, regardless of the severity of appendicitis (Grade A).

- Prophylactic drain placement cannot be advocated following simple cholecystectomy, either laparoscopic or open (Grade A).

- Prophylactic drain placement following liver resection is not beneficial and may even be detrimental (Grade A).

- Based on the available evidence, the routine placement of a T-tube following common bile duct exploration cannot be supported (Grade B). However, there may be a case for inserting a subhepatic drain for 24–48 h after closure of the common bile duct.

- In upper gastrointestinal and pancreatic surgery there is little evidence to support the use of drains.

- Currently, the placement of drains following incisional hernia repair has to be at the discretion of the operating surgeon.

- Percutaneous drainage is the recommended treatment for symptomatic postoperative collections and when there are signs of infection.

References

1. Robinson JO. Surgical drainage: an historical perspective. *Br J Surg* 1986; **73**: 422–426.
2. Iserson KV. J.F.B. Charrière: the man behind the 'French' gauge. *J Emerg Med* 1987; **5**: 545–548.
3. Public Health Laboratory Service. Incidence of surgical wound infection in England and Wales. *Lancet* 1960; **276**: 659–663.
4. Anon. Chapter IV. Factors influencing the incidence of wound infection. *Ann Surg* 1964; **160 (Suppl 2)**: 32–81.
5. Ngo QD, Lam VWT, Deane SA. *Drowning in Drainage: The Liverpool Hospital Survival Guide to Drains and Tubes.* Liverpool, NSW: Liverpool Hospital, 2004.
6. Meakins JL. Innovation in surgery: the rules of evidence. *Am J Surg* 2002; **183**: 399–405.
7. Cheatham ML, Chapman WC, Key SP, Sawyers JL. A meta-analysis of selective versus routine nasogastric decompression after elective laparotomy. *Ann Surg* 1995; **221**: 469–476.
8. Nelson R, Tse B, Edwards S. Systematic review of prophylactic nasogastric decompression after abdominal operations. *Br J Surg* 2005; **92**: 673–680.
9. Nelson R, Edwards S, Tse B. Prophylactic nasogastric decompression after abdominal surgery. Cochrane Database Syst Rev 2005;(1): CD004929.
10. Smith SR, Connolly JC, Crane PW, Gilmore OJ. The effect of surgical drainage materials on colonic healing. *Br J Surg* 1982; **69**: 153–155.
11. Karliczek A, Jesus EC, Matos D, Castro AA, Atallah AN, Wiggers T. Drainage or nondrainage in elective colorectal anastomosis: a systematic review and meta-analysis. *Colorectal Dis* 2006; **8**: 259–265.

12. Magarey CJ, Chant AD, Rickford CR, Magarey JR. Clinical trial of the effects of drainage and antibiotics after appendicectomy. *Br J Surg* 1971; **58**: 855–856.

13. Stone HH, Hooper CA, Millikan Jr WJ. Abdominal drainage following appendectomy and cholecystectomy. *Ann Surg* 1978; **187**: 606–612.

14. Dandapat MC, Panda C. A perforated appendix: should we drain? *J Indian Med Assoc* 1992; **90**: 147–148.

15. Greenall MJ, Evans M, Pollock AV. Should you drain a perforated appendix? *Br J Surg* 1978; **65**: 880–882.

16. Petrowsky H, Demartines N, Rousson V, Clavien PA. Evidence-based value of prophylactic drainage in gastrointestinal surgery: a systematic review and meta-analyses. *Ann Surg* 2004; **240**: 1074–1084.

17. Budd DC, Cochran RC, Fouty Jr WJ. Cholecystectomy with and without drainage. A randomized, prospective study of 300 patients. *Am J Surg* 1982; **143**: 307–309.

18. Monson JR, Guillou PJ, Keane FB, Tanner WA, Brennan TG. Cholecystectomy is safer without drainage: the results of a prospective, randomized clinical trial. *Surgery* 1991; **109**: 740–746.

19. Playforth MJ, Sauven P, Evans M, Pollock AV. Suction drainage of the gallbladder bed does not prevent complications after cholecystectomy: a random control clinical trial. *Br J Surg* 1985; **72**: 269–271.

20. Lewis RT, Goodall RG, Marien B, Park M, Lloyd-Smith W, Wiegand FM. Simple elective cholecystectomy: to drain or not. *Am J Surg* 1990; **159**: 241–245.

21. Gurusamy KS, Samraj K. Routine abdominal drainage for uncomplicated open cholecystectomy. Cochrane Database Syst Rev 2007;(2): CD006003.

22. Jorgensen JO, Gillies RB, Hunt DR, Caplehorn JR, Lumley T. A simple and effective way to reduce postoperative pain after laparoscopic cholecystectomy. *Aust NZ J Surg* 1995; **65**: 466–469.

23. Nursal TZ, Yildirim S, Tarim A *et al*. Effect of drainage on postoperative nausea, vomiting, and pain after laparoscopic cholecystectomy. *Langenbecks Arch Surg* 2003; **388**: 95–100.

24. Fong Y, Cohen AM, Fortner JG *et al*. Liver resection for colorectal metastases. *J Clin Oncol* 1997; **15**: 938–946.

25. Liu CL, Fan ST, Lo CM *et al*. Abdominal drainage after hepatic resection is contraindicated in patients with chronic liver diseases. *Ann Surg* 2004; **239**: 194–201.

26. Gurusamy KS, Samraj K, Davidson BR. Routine abdominal drainage for uncomplicated liver resection. Cochrane Database Syst Rev 2007;(3): CD006232.

27. De Roover D, Vanderveken M, Gerard Y. Choledochotomy: primary closure versus T-tube. A prospective trial. *Acta Chir Belg* 1989; **89**: 320–324.

28. Sheen-Chen SM, Chou FF. Choledochotomy for biliary lithiasis: is routine T-tube drainage necessary? A prospective controlled trial. *Acta Chir Scand* 1990; **156**: 387–390.

29. Williams JA, Treacy PJ, Sidey P, Worthley CS, Townsend NC, Russell EA. Primary duct closure versus T-tube drainage following exploration of the common bile duct. *Aust NZ J Surg* 1994; **64**: 823–826.

30. Pai D, Sharma A, Kanungo R, Jagdish S, Gupta A. Role of abdominal drains in perforated duodenal ulcer patients: a prospective controlled study. *Aust NZ J Surg* 1999; **69**: 210–213.

31. Kim J, Lee J, Hyung WJ *et al*. Gastric cancer surgery without drains: a prospective randomized trial. *J Gastrointest Surg* 2004; **8**: 727–732.

32. Kumar M, Yang SB, Jaiswal VK, Shah JN, Shreshtha M, Gongal R. Is prophylactic placement of drains necessary after subtotal gastrectomy? *World J Gastroenterol* 2007; **13**: 3738–3741.

33. Conlon KC, Labow D, Leung D *et al*. Prospective randomized clinical trial of the value of intraperitoneal drainage after pancreatic resection. *Ann Surg* 2001; **234**: 487–493.

34. Scevola S, Youssef A, Kroll SS, Langstein H. Drains and seromas in TRAM flap breast reconstruction. *Ann Plast Surg* 2002; **48**: 511–514.

35. George CD, Ellis H. The results of incisional hernia repair: a twelve year review. *Ann R Coll Surg Engl* 1986; **68**: 185–187.

36. White TJ, Santos MC, Thompson JS. Factors affecting wound complications in repair of ventral hernias. *Am Surg* 1998; **64**: 276–280.

37. Hesselink VJ, Luijendijk RW, de Wilt JH, Heide R, Jeekel J. An evaluation of risk factors in incisional hernia recurrence. *Surg Gynecol Obstet* 1993; **176**: 228–234.
38. Pessaux P, Msika S, Atalla D, Hay JM, Flamant Y. Risk factors for postoperative infectious complications in noncolorectal abdominal surgery: a multivariate analysis based on a prospective multicenter study of 4718 patients. *Arch Surg* 2003; **138**: 314–324.
39. Gurusamy KS, Samraj K. Wound drains after incisional hernia repair. Cochrane Database Syst Rev 2007;(1): CD005570.
40. Radder RW. Ultrasonically guided percutaneous catheter drainage for gallbladder empyema. *Diag Imaging* 1980; **49**: 330–333.
41. Hamy A, Visset J, Likholatnikov D *et al*. Percutaneous cholecystostomy for acute cholecystitis in critically ill patients. *Surgery* 1997; **121**: 398–401.
42. Spira RM, Nissan A, Zamir O, Cohen T, Fields SI, Freund HR. Percutaneous transhepatic cholecystostomy and delayed laparoscopic cholecystectomy in critically ill patients with acute calculus cholecystitis. *Am J Surg* 2002; **183**: 62–66.
43. Silberfein EJ, Zhou W, Kougias P *et al*. Percutaneous cholecystostomy for acute cholecystitis in high-risk patients: experience of a surgeon-initiated interventional program. *Am J Surg* 2007; **194**: 672–677.

Miguel A. Cuesta Donald van der Peet
Alexander Veenhof

3

Laparoscopic management of the acute abdomen

The acute abdomen is characterised by the sudden appearance of abdominal complaints that oblige the surgeon to decide promptly whether to operate immediately, to treat conservatively or to observe the patient.

In spite of new diagnostic developments, such as ultrasonography and computed tomography (CT), it seems that acute abdominal conditions present situations in which a surgeon dares to open an abdomen without a clear diagnosis. With the only exception of haemodynamic instability caused by the abdominal condition, this situation is changing in the surgical community: a proper pre-operative diagnosis can lead to better and more specific surgical treatment and to an improved approach.

In surgical practice, all acute abdominal situations can be divided into four categories: (i) local peritonitis, such as acute appendicitis or acute cholecystitis; (ii) perforation of a hollow organ such as duodenal ulcer with the presence of pneumoperitoneum; (iii) general peritonitis of uncertain aetiology, without perforation or intestinal obstruction, such as intestinal ischaemia; and (iv) intestinal obstruction.

After a full medical history and general and local physical examination, supplementary studies should be done including haematology, biochemistry and plain radiography of the abdomen. In most cases, the acute abdomen can then be diagnosed in one of the above mentioned diagnostic groups. Moreover,

Miguel A. Cuesta MD (for correspondence)
Professor of Gastro-intestinal Surgery, Department of Surgery, Academic Hospital Vrije Universiteit,
Post Box 7057, 1007 MB Amsterdam, The Netherlands. E-mail: ma.cuesta@vumc.nl

Donald van der Peet MD PhD
Department of Surgery, Academic Hospital Vrije Universiteit, Post Box 7057, 1007 MB Amsterdam,
The Netherlands

Alexander A.F.A. Veenhof MD
Department of Surgery, Academic Hospital Vrije Universiteit, Post Box 7057, 1007 MB Amsterdam,
The Netherlands

Table 1 Possibilities for initial diagnosis of the acute abdomen

- Localised peritonitis
  Acute cholecystitis
  Acute appendicitis (right lower abdomen)
  Acute diverticulitis
- Generalised peritonitis of unknown origin
- Peritonitis by perforation
  Perforated gastroduodenal ulcer
  Perforated acute diverticulitis (colon sigmoid)
- Intestinal obstruction

a clear diagnosis, if possible, is important in order to plan the right abdominal incision or to avoid an unnecessary laparotomy. Supplementary non-invasive procedures, such as ultrasonography or CT, are not always conclusive. Diagnostic laparoscopy is then the only technique which can visualise the abdominal cavity and, by establishing an adequate diagnosis, permit the surgeon to plan the right abdominal approach for the various possibilities listed in Table 1.

LOCALISED PERITONITIS

ACUTE CHOLECYSTITIS

Medical history and physical examination may indicate the diagnosis of acute cholecystitis. Ultrasonography will confirm the diagnosis. Typical findings on ultrasonography are increased size of the gallbladder with wall thickening with or without gallstones (calculous or acalculous cholecystitis) and, sometimes, the presence of fluid collections around the inflamed gallbladder. Ultrasonography will confirm the diagnosis with a very high sensitivity and specificity (gallbladder wall thickening has a sensitivity of 96%, specificity of 83% and an accuracy of 94%.[1]

Questions arise about when to operate for acute cholecystectomy by laparoscopy and what to do if the patient is not suitable for operation. Important points include the timing of surgery in relation to the interval from the onset of symptoms, the role of delayed laparoscopic cholecystectomy and the proper surgical technique. In order to decrease complications and to increase the success rate of laparoscopic cholecystectomy in acute cholecystitis, Gurusamy et al.[2] analysed all randomised studies performed in this area, and reported the benefits and harms. They compared early laparoscopic cholecystectomy (less than 7 days from onset of symptoms) versus delayed laparoscopic cholecystectomy (operated more than 6 weeks after index admission). Five trials were identified with 451 patients randomised – 223 to the early group and 228 to the delayed group. Surgery was performed on 222 patients in the early group and on 216 patients in the delayed group. There was no statistically significant difference between the two groups for any of the outcomes including bile duct injury and conversion to open cholecystectomy. A total of 40 patients (17.5%) from the delayed group had to undergo emergency laparoscopic cholecystectomy due to non-resolving or recurrent cholecystitis; 18 (45%) of these had to undergo conversion to open procedure. Moreover, total hospital stay was about 3 days shorter in the early group compared with the delayed group. Siddiqui *et al.*[3] and Lau *et al.*[4] confirmed this, and further analysis of the data did not show any significant differences between the two approaches in terms of operation time, conversion rate, overall complication rate, incidence of bile leakage, and intra-abdominal complications.[7,8] Early laparoscopic cholecystectomy during acute cholecystitis seems safe and cost-effective by shortening the total hospital stay.[3,4]

Concerning the timing of laparoscopic cholecystectomy in relation to the onset of symptoms, and the number of conversions and complications, Suter and Meyer[5] studied a group of 268 patients (151 women and 117 men), with a mean age of 53 years, who underwent surgery on an emergency basis for suspected acute cholecystitis. Delay before admission and surgery varied widely, but 72% of the patients underwent surgery within 48 h of admission. Intra-operative cholangiography, attempted in 218 patients, was successful in 207 (95%). Conversion was necessary in 15.6% of the cases. It occurred more frequently in patients who underwent surgery later than 48 h or 96 h after admission. No other predictor of conversion was found. Overall morbidity was 15.3%. Three partial lesions of the common bile duct occurred. All were recognised and repaired immediately. In experienced hands, laparoscopic cholecystectomy, performed within 2, or at most 4, days of admission, is safe, effective and is the treatment of choice for acute cholecystitis. Intra-operative cholangiography should be performed in every case because it helps to clarify the anatomy and allows for early diagnosis and repair of bile duct injuries.[5]

Exceptions to this approach may be patients who are critically ill (ASA III or IV) or high-risk elderly patients in whom the operation is likely to cause morbidity and mortality. Percutaneous transhepatic cholecystostomy (PTCh) may be the proper initial approach before a laparoscopic cholecystectomy can be performed with the patient in a better general condition. Spira *et al.*[6] studied the role of PTCh and delayed laparoscopic cholecystostomy in critically ill patients with acute cholecystitis. They reviewed 55 patients who underwent PTCh. The main indications in these high-risk patients were biliary sepsis and septic shock in 23 patients (42%) and severe co-morbidities in 32 patients (58%). The median age was 74 years (range, 32–98 years); there were 33 women and 22 men. Successful biliary drainage by PTCh was achieved in 54 of 55 (98%) of the patients. The majority of the patients (31 of 55) were drained transhepatically under CT guidance and the rest were drained using ultrasound guidance followed by cholecystography for verification. Complications included hepatic bleeding that required surgical intervention in one patient and dislodgement of the catheter in 9 patients that was reinserted in 2 patients. Three patients died of multi-organ failure. The remaining 52 patients recovered well with a mean hospital stay of 15.5 ± 11.4 days. Thirty-one patients were able to undergo delayed surgery: 28 underwent laparoscopic cholecystectomy of whom 4 (14%) were converted to open cholecystectomy.[6] Percutaneous transhepatic cholecystostomy is a valuable and effective procedure in a high-risk group of patients with acute cholecystitis. Due to the high co-morbidity of the patient population the procedure has a high morbidity and mortality. It should be considered, with exceptions, as a bridge to elective cholecystectomy.

Key point 1

- Percutaneous transhepatic cholecystostomy is a valuable and effective procedure in a high-risk group of patients with acute cholecystitis.

Technique of acute laparoscopic cholecystectomy

The position of the patient and placement of trocars will be the same as for elective laparoscopic cholecystectomy. Four trocars are introduced, under the umbilicus for the laparoscope and the other three for instruments, under the costal margin (Fig. 1). If there is significant distention, the gallbladder should be aspirated immediately. The safety principles of the critical view, as defined by Strasberg et al.,[7] should be adopted in order to avoid injury to the common bile duct (CBD). Depending on the grade of inflammation, the gallbladder can

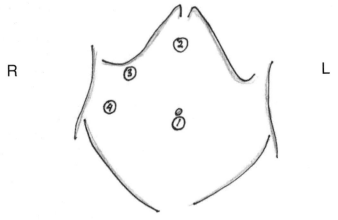

Fig. 1 Placement of cannulas for laparoscopic cholecystectomy.

be dissected from the triangle of Calot to the fundus (routine cholecystectomy), or retrogradely (fundus-first cholecystectomy) if visualisation is difficult in the triangle. Blunt, careful dissection by an experienced surgeon will be key to success. In more difficult cases, a partial cholecystectomy can be performed, after retrieving all stones, leaving a small part of the gallbladder or the posterior wall behind. Routine peri-operative cholangiography may be advisable.

Conversion will be performed early during the procedure if there is no progression to identification of anatomy or when there is continuous bleeding.

In conclusion, early laparoscopic cholecystectomy is the treatment of choice in patients with acute cholecystitis with acceptable risk. Experience probably reduces the number of conversions. Exceptions to this will be the high-risk patient group (ASA III or IV patients), the presence of a palpable phlegmon, previous upper abdominal laparotomy, presence of obstructive jaundice or coagulation problems. The possibility of temporary treatment of sepsis by percutaneous transhepatic drainage should be considered after correction of coagulation. Whenever possible, a delayed, elective, laparoscopic cholecystectomy should be planned.

Key point 2

- Early laparoscopic cholecystectomy is the treatment of choice in patients with acute cholecystitis with acceptable risk.

ACUTE APPENDICITIS (RIGHT LOWER ABDOMEN PERITONITIS)

Physical examination and medical history remain the most important steps in patients with acute right lower quadrant abdominal pain. White blood cell (WBC) count and serum C-reactive protein (CRP) may be helpful. Urinary sediment examination and pregnancy tests should be undertaken when necessary. Andersson et al.[8] reported the diagnostic value of medical history, clinical presentation and indices of inflammation in a group of 496 patients with suspected acute appendicitis. None of the individual variables had sufficiently high discriminating power to be used as diagnostic test. Leukocyte and WBC counts, CRP, rebound tenderness, and gender were independent predictors of appendicitis.[8] A meta-analysis of studies addressing these issues has shown increased likelihood of appendicitis when fever or pain migrating to the lower abdomen and a positive psoas sign were present.[9] Bohner et al.[10] showed a maximum positive predictive value of 85% when a combination of three out of five clinical parameters were present.

Combining clinical history, physical examination and laboratory studies has led to the development of scoring systems and computer-aided algorithms to help clinicians with decision making in acute appendicitis.[11] Overall, the actual gain of scoring systems appears small and the performance of these scores outside study conditions is often disappointing. Ohmann et al.[12] studied in 1254 patients with suspected appendicitis, using ten different scores and found that none of the scores fulfilled any of the performance criteria determined beforehand.

Imaging techniques

Several imaging techniques have been advocated to improve diagnostic accuracy in patients with suspected acute appendicitis. Rao et al.[13] evaluated plain abdominal radiography. No individual finding on the plain abdominal radiograph was sensitive or specific. Plain radiography should not be obtained routinely in such patients.[13]

The value of pre-operative ultrasonography has been demonstrated in numerous studies. Puylaert et al.[14] showed a specificity of 100% and a much lower sensitivity of 75% for ultrasonography in patients with suspected acute appendicitis. In patients with perforated appendicitis, the sensitivity was notably low (28.5%). More recently, Allemann et al.[15] showed a specificity of 99% and sensitivity of 91% in these patients. However, ultrasonography has a high inter- and intra-observer variability, being more difficult in patients with a body mass index exceeding 25 kg/m^2. In a meta-analysis by Orr et al.,[16] which included 17 studies and a total of 3358 patients, overall sensitivity and specificity of ultrasonography were 85% and 92%, respectively. In this study, ultrasonography proved most useful for patients with intermediate probability of appendicitis, based upon clinical examination.[16] There is growing evidence that CT may be superior to ultrasonography in diagnosing acute appendicitis. Although CT has the disadvantage of exposing the patient to radiation, its consistent sensitivity and specificity of over 90% in many studies, and the low inter- and intra-observer variability, may make CT the optimal non-invasive diagnostic procedure in a patient with suspected appendicitis. Rao et al.,[17] in a recent study demonstrated that routine CT in these patients resulted in improved patient care and reduced use of hospital resources. Wise et al.[18] recommended a standard unenhanced abdominopelvic CT as the initial examination. Poortman et al.[19] performed a radiologist-blinded prospective study on 199 consecutive patients examined with ultrasonography and CT. All patients were operated on: 132 patients had acute appendicitis at surgery and 67 patients did not. Sensitivity of CT and ultrasonography was 76% and 79%, respectively; specificity was 83% and 78%, accuracy 78% and 78%, with positive predictive values 90% and 87%, respectively. Their conclusion was that unenhanced helical CT and graded compression ultrasonography by radiologists have a similar accuracy for the diagnosis of acute appendicitis.[19]

Key point 3

- Helical computed tomography or an ultrasonography performed by a radiologist will resolve the diagnosis in many patients with right iliac fossa pain.

Diagnostic laparoscopy

Laparoscopic inspection of the abdominal cavity enables the surgeon to diagnose acute appendicitis accurately. Moreover, it has been showed that leaving an appendix that appears normal during laparoscopic inspection is safe.[20] Criteria for the diagnosis of appendicitis during laparoscopic inspection are the presence of unequivocal inflammatory changes, such as pus, fibrin, or vascular injection of the serosa. Rigidity and lack of mobility at manipulation are less certain signs of inflammation.

Removing a normal appendix at open surgery is associated with a 7–13% risk of early complications and 4% of late complication such as incisional hernia and chronic pain in the first year after operation. If a normal appendix is left *in situ* during diagnostic laparoscopy, the number of unnecessary appendicectomies will decrease, particularly in fertile women (17–45%). The diagnostic yield of laparoscopy in patients with suspected appendicitis is high, but laparoscopy may be considered too invasive to justify its use only for diagnostic purposes. This reasoning seems particularly true in the era of helical CT.

Before the routine use of ultrasonography or CT, and to establish the place of diagnostic laparoscopy in our department, a study was conducted in 1999 to determine the value of diagnostic laparoscopy in fertile women in order to reduce the number of negative appendicectomies and establish the correct diagnosis to allow prompt and appropriate treatment.[21]

A total of 161 consecutive adult female patients under 50 years of age with a clinical diagnosis of acute appendicitis underwent diagnostic laparoscopy prior to the planned appendicectomy. Other diagnoses were treated accordingly. A normal appendix was not removed. Results were compared to a group of 23 postmenopausal women, and to all 137 male adults. After laparoscopy, 55% of the patients required appendicectomy for appendicitis while in 23% a gynaecological diagnosis was made in spite of previous examination by a gynaecologist. Fourteen percent had a negative laparoscopy. There were no false-negative results. The respective rates of negative laparoscopy for postmenopausal women and men were 4% and 8%, respectively. We concluded, after this study, that all women of fertile age suspected of having acute appendicitis should undergo diagnostic laparoscopy prior to the planned appendicectomy, regardless of the certainty of the pre-operative diagnosis. This is currently the only way to reduce the negative appendicectomy rate and establish a correct diagnosis allowing prompt and appropriate treatment. In male patients and postmenopausal women with local peritonitis of the lower abdomen, the diagnosis is acute appendicitis in more than 90% of cases.

Even after the extended use of ultrasonography (and CT) in all patients suspected of having acute appendicitis, around 20% of female patients and 8–10% of male patients will have a negative appendix during laparoscopic intervention. Therefore, in all patients planned to undergo a laparoscopic appendicectomy, the initial diagnostic character of this intervention should be stressed. If the appendix is normal, the whole abdominal cavity should be examined, starting with the internal genitals.

Cochrane Central Register

Sauerland et al.[22] looked at the diagnostic and therapeutic effects of laparoscopic and conventional 'open' surgery in the Cochrane Central Register of Controlled Trials. They included randomised clinical trials comparing laparoscopic (LA) versus open appendectomy (OA) in adults or children. Fifty-four studies, of which 45 compared LA (with or without diagnostic laparoscopy) versus OA in adults were included. Wound infections were less likely after LA than after OA (OR 0.45; 95% CI 0.35–0.58), but the incidence of intra-abdominal abscesses was increased (OR 2.48; 95% CI 1.45–4.21). The duration of surgery was 12 min (95% CI 7–16) longer for LA. Pain on day 1 after surgery was reduced after LA by 9 mm (95% CI 5–13 mm) on a 100 mm visual analogue scale. Hospital stay was shortened by 1.1 days (95% CI 0.6 to 1.5). Return to normal activity, work, and sport occurred earlier after LA than after OA. While the operation costs of LA were significantly higher, the costs outside hospital were reduced. Five studies on children were included, but the results do not seem to be much different when compared to adults. Diagnostic laparoscopy reduced the risk of a negative appendectomy, but this effect was stronger in fertile women (RR 0.20; 95% CI 0.11–0.34) compared to unselected adults (RR 0.37; 95% CI 0.13–1.01). In those clinical settings where surgical expertise and equipment are available and affordable, diagnostic laparoscopy and LA (either in combination or separately) seem to have various advantages over OA. Some of the clinical effects of LA, however, are small and of limited clinical relevance. Laparoscopy and LA are generally recommended in patients with suspected appendicitis unless laparoscopy itself is contra-indicated or not feasible. Young female, obese, and employed patients seem to benefit especially from LA.

Operative technique

A zero degree 10-mm laparoscope is introduced through an infra-umbilical incision in order to inspect the abdominal cavity. Another 5 mm cannula is introduced cranial to the pubic bone in the midline (Fig. 2). The first step is the identification of the appendix. Inspection of the appendix involves assessment of colour, consistency, mobility, fixation and possible perforation. When the appendix is located posterior to the caecum, this should be mobilised first by cutting the peritoneum at Told's line. This is facilitated by introducing a third cannula just medial to the left anterior superior iliac spine. If the appendix appears normal, the gallbladder, stomach, duodenum, sigmoid colon, small bowel, and internal genitals are inspected. A normal appendix should be left *in situ*.

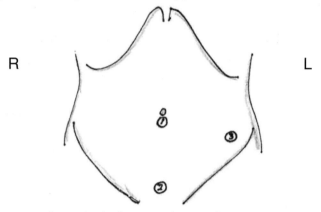

R   L

Fig. 2 Placement of cannulas for laparoscopic appendicectomy.

In the majority of cases, retrograde dissection of the appendix (base to tip) is preferred, only dense infiltration of the base may require antegrade dissection. The meso-appendix is skeletonised once the appendix is retracted by means of a grasper. The meso-appendix is skeletonised to expose the appendicular artery, using monopolar diathermy, clips or an ultrasonic device. The appendix must be completely dissected in order to avoid a partial appendicectomy. The appendix stump can be ligated with pre-tied loops at the base of appendix (two left and one on the removed side). Transection of the appendix between loops must be done carefully in order to avoid tearing of the loops. If the base of the appendix is infiltrated, or the base perforated, the appendicectomy will be performed using a stapling device (blue cartridge, 30 mm) across the healthy base or even on the caecum. The use of a stapling device is mandatory when there is a perforation at the base of the appendix.

The appendix is removed through the widest cannula; when the passage of the appendix through the cannula is unlikely, the appendix is placed in a

Key point 4

- All patients suspected of acute appendicitis should have an ultrasonography. Patients will be clinically divided in equivocal and unequivocal acute appendicitis.

plastic retrieval bag prior to removal. Suction is performed routinely to remove blood, purulent material, *etc*. If there are abscesses or general peritonitis, the abdominal cavity should be irrigated and cleaned by means of lavage with saline. No drain is left behind.

Key point 5–7

- Unequivocal clinical diagnosis plus positive ultrasonography will require diagnostic laparoscopy followed by laparoscopic appendicectomy.

- Unequivocal clinical diagnosis plus negative ultrasonography will lead to clinical observation. A helical computed tomography should be done to exclude other diagnoses. If the clinical condition worsens, a diagnostic laparoscopy should be performed.

- An equivocal diagnosis will lead to clinical (at home) observation. If local peritoneal signs develop, a diagnostic laparoscopy should be performed.

GENERAL PERITONITIS

There are acute abdominal conditions in which it is difficult to establish a diagnosis before laparotomy. A diagnosis is important in planning the right abdominal incision or to avoid an unnecessary laparotomy. Non-invasive diagnostic procedures such as plain abdominal X-ray, ultrasonography or CT are not always conclusive. Diagnostic laparoscopy is the only technique which can visualise the abdomen and, by establishing an adequate diagnosis, permit the surgeon to plan the right abdominal approach. In our department, a prospective study was performed in 65 patients with a generalised acute abdomen (with no signs of intestinal obstruction or perforation on plain X-ray and ultrasonography). All the patients underwent diagnostic laparoscopy under general anaesthesia before the planned exploratory laparotomy. In 46 patients (70%), diagnostic laparoscopy permitted the establishment of an adequate diagnosis, whereas in seven patients (10%) no cause for the acute abdomen could be found and an exploratory laparotomy was avoided. In another 12 patients (20%), insufficient information was obtained during laparoscopy and an exploratory laparotomy was performed. A conclusive diagnosis was established in 53 patients. Information from laparoscopy led to a change in the surgical approach in 38 patients (*e.g.* limited, well-placed approach, laparoscopic surgery, or avoidance of an unnecessary laparotomy). Diagnostic laparoscopy in this category of patients is a useful technique with important therapeutic consequences.[23]

TECHNIQUE OF DIAGNOSTIC LAPAROSCOPY

Diagnostic laparoscopy is done under general anaesthesia. Prophylactic antibiotics are administered intravenously and the urinary bladder is catheterised. A three-port approach is generally used (Fig. 3): infra-umbilical

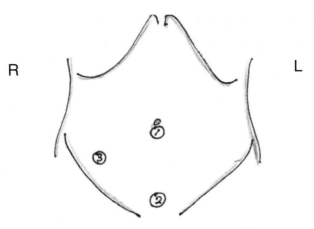

Fig. 3 Placement of cannulas for diagnostic laparoscopy and lavage.

(laparoscope); suprapubic (5 mm); and the right abdomen, lateral to the umbilicus (5 mm). By adjusting the operating table, the position of the patient can be changed and the abdomen can be explored adequately. Pus or other fluids can be seen easily, particularly in the pouch of Douglas, paracolic gutters, and subphrenic and subhepatic spaces. This can be aspirated for laboratory tests. In this way, the liver and gallbladder, stomach and duodenum, appendix and internal genital organs, small intestine and colon are all adequately visualised.

In patients with symptoms of acute abdomen with no specific localisation, a mid-line laparotomy is the classical approach in order to establish a diagnosis and to treat the problem. Using this approach, the surgeon frequently comes to the conclusion that the incision was too long (*e.g.* starting with an upper median laparotomy and finding a perforated appendix), or misplaced (starting with a McBurney incision to approach the appendix and finding a perforated duodenal ulcer). In other patients, the cause of the problem could have been treated conservatively or laparoscopically. The advantage of a well-chosen approach is not only cosmetic but also the decrease in operative trauma, which will also reduce frequent wound infections as well as the resulting incisional hernias.

Laparoscopy is the only exploration that can directly visualise the abdominal cavity and diagnose peritonitis because of the presence of fluids in paracolic gutters and the pouch of Douglas, and subphrenic and subhepatic abscesses. Moreover, it can visualise the affected organ, indicating the best surgical approach to solve the problem. In some cases, laparoscopy will help to avoid an unnecessary laparotomy; for example, if there is mesenteric ischaemia with necrosis. If the diagnostic laparoscopy is negative and depending on the experience of the surgeon, unnecessary laparotomy can be avoided.

Key point 8

- Diagnostic laparoscopy should be performed in all patients with signs of a generalised acute abdomen in whom no clear cause is suspected after clinical, radiological and laboratory investigation. A correct diagnosis will dictate the right surgical approach.

PERITONITIS BY PERFORATION

Medical history and physical examination are the cornerstones in the diagnosis of generalised peritonitis. On plain X-ray, the presence of pneumoperitoneum will confirm perforation of a hollow organ as the cause of the peritonitis. In practice, there are two main possibilities (with many other scenarios) – a perforated gastroduodenal ulcer or perforated diverticulitis of the sigmoid colon.

Symptoms are important to help differentiate between them. Symptoms initiated in the upper abdomen, and a history of chronic pain or the use of NSAIDs, will favour the diagnosis of perforated ulcer whereas symptoms initiated in the lower abdomen will favour the diagnosis of perforated diverticulitis.

If suspicion exists of perforated diverticulitis, an enhanced CT should be done.

Diagnostic laparoscopy will differentiate the type of perforation and guide the surgical treatment.

PERFORATED GASTRODUODENAL ULCER

In the case of perforated ulcers, mostly duodenal, different methods have been used to close the perforated ulcer. Closure by stitches with or without omentoplasty, or sutureless closure by omentum are the usual techniques used.

Because the clinical condition of patients is so variable, only haemodynamically stable patients are candidates for laparoscopic approach. Haemodynamic instability is a contra-indication for laparoscopy because delay can worsen the condition of the patient.

To compare the outcome of patients operated either laparoscopically or open, there are two randomised studies, two meta-analyses, and one Cochrane review. Lau et al.[24] studied 103 patients with juxtapyloric and duodenal ulcers who were randomly allocated to laparoscopic suture repair, laparoscopic sutureless repair, open suture repair, and open sutureless repair. Laparoscopic repair of perforated peptic ulcer (groups 1 and 2) took significantly longer than open repair (groups 3 and 4; 94.3 ± 40.3 min versus 53.7 ± 42.6 min) but the amount of analgesic required after laparoscopic repair was significantly less than in open surgery. There was no significant difference in the four groups of patients in terms of duration of nasogastric aspiration, duration of intravenous drip, total hospital stay, time to resume normal diet, visual analogue scale score for pain in the first 24 h after surgery, morbidity, re-operation, and mortality rates. They concluded that laparoscopic repair of perforated peptic ulcer is a viable option. Sutureless repair is as safe as suture repair and it takes less time to perform.[24]

Siu et al.[25] randomised 130 patients with a clinical diagnosis of perforated peptic ulcer to undergo either open or laparoscopic omental patch repair. Laparoscopic repair was converted to an open procedure for technical difficulties, non-juxtapyloric gastric ulcers, or perforations larger than 10 mm. Nine patients with a surgical diagnosis other than perforated peptic ulcer were excluded; 121 patients entered the final analysis. There were 98 male and 23 female patients recruited, aged 16–89 years. There were nine conversions in the laparoscopic group. After surgery, patients in the laparoscopic group required significantly less parenteral analgesics than those who underwent open repair, and the visual analogue pain scores on days 1 and 3 after surgery were significantly lower in the laparoscopic group. Laparoscopic repair required significantly less time than open repair. The median postoperative stay was 6 days in the laparoscopic group versus 7 days in the open group. There were fewer chest infections in the laparoscopic group. There were two intra-abdominal collections in the laparoscopic group. One patient in the laparoscopic group and three patients in the open group died after surgery. Laparoscopic repair of perforated peptic ulcer is considered a safe and reliable procedure. It was associated with a shorter operating time, less postoperative pain, reduced chest complications, a shorter postoperative hospital stay, and earlier return to normal daily activities than the conventional open repair.[25]

The meta-analysis performed by Lau[26] in 2004 of 13 studies suggests that laparoscopic repair of perforated peptic ulcer confers superior short-term benefits in terms of postoperative pain and wound morbidity. This approach is as safe and effective as open repair.[26] The review performed recently by Lunevicius et al.,[27] of 15 well-performed studies, concluded that laparoscopic repair seems better than open repair for low-risk patients. However, limited knowledge about its benefits and risks compared with open repair suggests that the latter, more familiar, approach may be more appropriate in high-risk patients. Statistically significant findings in favour of laparoscopic repair were less analgesic use, shorter hospital stay, less wound infection and lower mortality rate. Shorter operating time and less suture-site leakage were advantages of open repair. Three variables (hospital stay, operating time and analgesic use) were significantly heterogeneous in the papers analysed.[27]

The Cochrane systemic review performed by Sanabria et al.[28] on the two above mentioned studies suggests that a decrease in septic abdominal complications may exist when laparoscopic surgery is used to correct perforated peptic ulcer. However, it is necessary to develop more randomised controlled trials that include a greater number of patients to confirm such an assumption, guaranteeing a long learning curve for participating surgeons.[28]

Key point 9

- Laparoscopic closure of perforated duodenal ulcer, in experienced hands, confers superior short-term benefits in terms of postoperative pain and wound morbidity.

Operative technique

Under general anaesthesia and prophylactic antibiotics, the abdomen is insufflated through an incision below the umbilicus. Four cannulas are used: a 30° laparoscope is introduced under the umbilicus and the other three cannulas (one of 10 mm and two of 5 mm) are placed between the left subcostal margin and the umbilicus, under the xyphoid and right lateral of the umbilicus (Fig. 4). After inspection of the abdominal cavity, the liver should be displaced

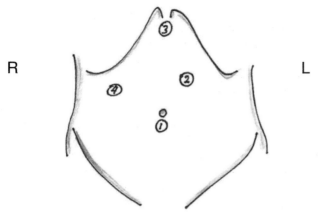

Fig. 4 Placement of cannulas for closure of duodenal ulcer perforation.

from the post-pyloric area to demonstrate the perforation. Fibrin and fluid collections will be removed and aspirated. If there is doubt, methylene-blue instillation through the nasogastric tube will identify the perforation. If no duodenal ulcer perforation is found, the rest of the abdominal cavity should be extensively inspected. It is important to inspect the lesser sac, in case there is a perforated posterior gastric ulcer. In order to visualise the lesser sac and the posterior gastric wall, the gastrocolic ligament should be opened. If there is an ulcer here, conversion to laparotomy is indicated. In gastric ulcer, biopsies should be taken to rule out gastric adenocarcinoma. A duodenal perforation should be closed using one or two stitches (Vicryl, 3-0), reinforced by omentoplasty. Saline lavage of the abdominal cavity should be performed. Usually no drain is needed.

PERFORATED DIVERTICULITIS

The current standard approach for perforated diverticulitis is open surgery. In selected patients with purulent peritonitis (Hinchey grade 3), a resection of the sigmoid can be followed by a primary anastomosis; however, in faecal peritonitis (Hinchey grade 4), the most frequent intervention is the Hartmann procedure.[29] A high morbidity and mortality are associated with this open approach. In 1996, O'Sullivan et al.[30] described eight patients who had peritoneal lavage alone as treatment for Hinchey grade 3 peritonitis with very good results and no recurrence after 3 years. Using the same laparoscopic lavage, Myers et al.[31] reported a prospective multi-institutional study on the role of laparoscopic surgery in 100 patients with perforated diverticulitis of the sigmoid colon, including 25 patients with Hinchey grade 2, 67 patients with grade 3, and 8 patients with grade 4. After confirmation of the diagnosis by plain X-ray and/or CT, patients were stabilised and then operated on. Hartmann's procedure was performed for faecal peritonitis. If purulent peritonitis was found, patients underwent peritoneal lavage in all four quadrants using 4 l or more of warmed saline until drainage was clear. Two Penrose drains were placed. Antibiotics were given for a week. The 92 patients with grades 2 or 3 peritonitis were managed by peritoneal lavage with morbidity and mortality rates of 4% and 3%, respectively. No resolution after laparoscopic lavage led to two patients having a Hartmann procedure and two others had intervention for pelvic abscess. Complete resolution was achieved in 87 patients. Only two patients re-presented with diverticulitis at a median follow-up of 36 months. Laparoscopic lavage and drainage in the acute management of perforated acute diverticulitis may be a promising alternative to more radical procedures, including the Hartmann's procedure. Acute resection should still be carried out in patients found to have faecal peritonitis or who fail to improve following lavage.

Key point 10

- Laparoscopic lavage and drainage in the acute management of perforated acute diverticulitis is a promising alternative to more radical procedures.

INTESTINAL OBSTRUCTION

In the evaluation of the patient presenting with intestinal obstruction, medical history and physical examination are important to establish the diagnosis and treatment. A plain X-ray of the abdomen in erect and supine positions will give important information about the type of obstruction, small or large bowel obstruction and the approximate localisation of the obstruction. CT will give additional information about the presence of a tumour or phlegmon and characterise a perforation better. Laparoscopy may be used, for treatment of an intestinal obstruction.

INDICATIONS FOR LAPAROSCOPY

The presence of a band or adhesions is the most frequent cause of small intestinal obstruction in a previously operated patient. Other causes are the presence of an incarcerated inguinal (or femoral) hernia or an obstructive tumour in the caecum. If the patient has never been operated and has no hernias, an internal hernia (with volvulus) or tumour will be the most frequent diagnosis. Bands and internal hernias or small bowel tumours may be approached laparoscopically. In the case of obstruction of the colon, a colonoscopy or an enema will give information about the localisation and the character of the obstruction, mostly a colon cancer. Laparoscopy for colon cancer with obstruction is very difficult due to the large dilatation of the proximal colon. These tumours, mostly distally located in the descending colon, sigmoid or rectosigmoid junction, can nowadays be stented. After a few days, the distention of the proximal colon disappears and the tumour can be resected laparoscopically.[32]

IS LAPAROSCOPY POSSIBLE IN AN INTESTINAL OBSTRUCTION?

Of course, the general contra-indications for a laparoscopic procedure also apply in the patients with intestinal obstruction. Distension of the bowel occupies space in the abdomen, the virtual expandable space is limited. Furthermore, the introduction of the first cannula can be hazardous and needs special care. An open introduction method should always be used. The presence of an abscess or pus is not a contra-indication for a laparoscopic procedure. A high conversion rate seems inevitable in this complex patient category, as is outlined in several studies. However, with growing experience in laparoscopic surgery this rate may decline.[33] So, if a laparoscopy is indicated and seems possible, how should it be done?

POSITIONING OF PATIENT AND CANNULAS

Depending of the expected findings at laparoscopy, the patient can be positioned accordingly. If a left colon resection has to be done, the patient should be placed in stirrups in order to facilitate a distal anastomosis using a circular stapler. In most other cases, no such specific position is necessary. The umbilicus is the preferred location for the open introduction of the first cannula (11 mm). The other cannulas can be placed according to the findings at laparoscopy. Extra cannulas should vary in size between 5–12 mm depending on the kind of procedure that is necessary. In general, most stapling devices need a 12- mm port and most haemostatic devices can be used through a 10-mm trocar.

EVIDENCE FOR THE LAPAROSCOPIC APPROACH IN INTESTINAL OBSTRUCTION

In the European Association for Endoscopic Surgery consensus statement on laparoscopy for abdominal emergencies, Sauerland et al.[34] give an evidence-based guideline on this subject. Although the patient presenting with intestinal obstruction is not explicitly mentioned, their paragraph on small bowel obstruction due to adhesions addresses this topic. The increased risk of bowel injury and the high conversion rates are mentioned. Ghosheh et al.[35] performed an extended search in the literature (Medline database) using the key words laparoscopy and bowel obstruction. Studies that included patients with chronic abdominal pain, chronic recurrent small bowel obstruction, or gastric or colonic obstruction were excluded. Nineteen studies between 1994 and 2005 were identified. Laparoscopy was attempted in 1061 patients with acute small bowel obstruction. The most common aetiologies of obstruction included adhesions (83.2%), abdominal wall hernia (3.1%), malignancy (2.9%), internal hernia (1.9%), and bezoars (0.8%). Laparoscopic treatment was possible in 705 cases with a conversion rate to open surgery of 33.5%. Causes of conversion were dense adhesions (27.7%), the need for bowel resection (23.1%), unidentified aetiology (13.0%), iatrogenic injury (10.2%), malignancy (7.4%), inadequate visualisation (4.2%), hernia (3.2%), and other causes (11.1%). Morbidity was 15.5% (152 of 981 patients) and mortality was 1.5% (16 of 1046 patients). There were 45 recognised intra-operative enterotomies (6.5%), but less than half resulted in conversion. There were, however, nine missed perforations, including one trocar injury, often resulting in significant morbidity. Early (within 30 days of surgery) recurrence of symptoms occurred in 2.1% of cases. Their conclusion was that laparoscopy is an effective procedure for the treatment of acute small bowel obstruction with acceptable risk of morbidity and early recurrence.

Levard et al.[36] studied 308 patients with acute small bowel obstruction treated laparoscopically in 35 centres. Conversion to laparotomy was accomplished in 140 patients (45.4%), during the same operation in 126 patients and after a median delay of 4 days (range, 1–12 days) in 14 patients. There were significantly more successes in patients with a history of one or two surgical interventions than in those with more than two (56% versus 37%; $P <$ 0.05). Moreover, there were significantly more successes in patients who had previously undergone an appendicectomy as cause of the obstruction (67 of 94; 71%). The rate of success was significantly higher ($P < 0.001$) in patients operated on early (< 24 h) and in patients with bands (54%), than in those with adhesions (31%) or with other causes of obstruction (15%). The median duration of postoperative ileus was significantly shorter in the 'success' group than in the 'failure' group (2 days versus 4 days; $P < 0.001$). The median duration of postoperative hospital stay was shorter in the 'success' group than in the 'failure' group (4 days versus 10 days; $P < 0.001$). The total number of immediate or delayed complications and particularly the number of recurrent obstructions after hospitalisation as well as the number of deaths did not differ significantly between the two groups.

Key point 11

- Laparoscopy is an effective procedure for the treatment of acute small bowel obstruction with acceptable risk of morbidity and early recurrence, but conversion rates of 30–40% should be expected.

SELECTION FOR LAPAROSCOPY

Whether to use the laparoscopic approach for intestinal obstruction is a difficult decision. There is a group of patients in whom a laparoscopic approach can be done with high possibility of conversion. Obstructed left colon treated previously by stent and decompression seems a relative good indication for a planned laparoscopic colon intervention. Moreover, a previously unoperated patient with small bowel obstruction (and without external hernias) may also be approached by laparoscopy. The value of laparoscopy for the most frequent patient, with laparotomy in the past, with intestinal obstruction as consequence of bands or adhesions is difficult to ascertain. The best candidates for success are patients with only one or two previous operations, especially appendicectomy or gynaecological interventions. Conversion remains around 40% with high possibility of enterostomies, recognised or not. A careful approach and randomised studies are necessary. With growing experience and strict indications a laparoscopy seems sound practice in the work-up of the patient with intestinal obstruction.

Key points for clinical practice

- Percutaneous transhepatic cholecystostomy is a valuable and effective procedure in a high-risk group of patients with acute cholecystitis.

- Early laparoscopic cholecystectomy is the treatment of choice in patients with acute cholecystitis with acceptable risk.

- Helical computed tomography or an ultrasonography performed by a radiologist will resolve the diagnosis in many patients with right iliac fossa pain.

- All patients suspected of acute appendicitis should have an ultrasonography. Patients will be clinically divided in equivocal and unequivocal acute appendicitis.

- Unequivocal clinical diagnosis plus positive ultrasonography will require diagnostic laparoscopy followed by laparoscopic appendicectomy.

- Unequivocal clinical diagnosis plus negative ultrasonography will lead to clinical observation. A helical computed tomography should be done to exclude other diagnoses. If the clinical condition worsens, a diagnostic laparoscopy should be performed.

- An equivocal diagnosis will lead to clinical (at home) observation. If local peritoneal signs develop, a diagnostic laparoscopy should be performed.

- Diagnostic laparoscopy should be performed in all patients with signs of a generalised acute abdomen in whom no clear cause is suspected after clinical, radiological and laboratory investigation. A correct diagnosis will dictate the right surgical approach.

- Laparoscopic closure of perforated duodenal ulcer, in experienced hands, confers superior short-term benefits in terms of postoperative pain and wound morbidity.

- Laparoscopic lavage and drainage in the acute management of perforated acute diverticulitis is a promising alternative to more radical procedures.

- Laparoscopy is an effective procedure for the treatment of acute small bowel obstruction with acceptable risk of morbidity and early recurrence, but conversion rates of 30–40% should be expected.

References

1. Park MS, Yu JS, Kim YH *et al*. Acute cholecystitis: comparison of MR, cholangiography and US. *Radiology* 1998; **209**: 781–785.
2. Gurusamy KS, Samraj K. Early versus delayed laparoscopic cholecystectomy for acute cholecystitis: a meta-analysis of randomized clinical trials. Cochrane Database Syst Rev 2006; (4) CD005440.
3. Siddiqui T, MacDonald A, Chong PS *et al*. Early versus delayed laparoscopic

cholecystectomy for acute cholecystitis: a meta-analysis of randomized clinical trials. *Am J Surg* 2008; **195**: 40–47.

4. Lau H, Lo CY, Patil NG *et al*. Early versus delayed-interval laparoscopic cholecystectomy for acute cholecystitis: a meta-analysis. *Surg Endosc* 2006; **20**: 82–87.

5. Suter M, Meyer A. A 10-year experience with the use of laparoscopic cholecystectomy for acute cholecystitis: is it safe? *Surg Endosc* 2001; **15**: 1187–1192.

6. Spira RM, Nissan A, Zamir O *et al*. Percutaneous trans-hepatic cholecystostomy and delayed laparoscopic cholecystectomy in critically ill patients with acute cholecystitis. *Am J Surg* 2002; **183**: 62–66.

7. Strasberg SM, Hertl M, Soper NJ. An analysis of the problem of biliary injury during laparoscopic cholecystectomy. *J Am Coll Surg* 1995; **180**: 101–125.

8. Andersson RE, Hugander AP, Ghazi SH *et al*. Why does the clinical diagnosis fail in suspected appendicitis? *Eur J Surg* 2000; **166**: 796–802.

9. Wagner JM, McKinney WP, Carpenter JL. Does this patient have appendicitis? *JAMA* 1996; **276**: 1589–1594.

10. Bohner H, Yang Q, Franke K *et al*. Significance of anamnesis and clinical findings for diagnosis of acute appendicitis. Acute Abdominal Pain Study Group. *Z Gastroenterol* 1994; **32**: 579–583.

11. De Dombal FT, Dallos V, McAdam WA. Can computer aided teaching packages improve clinical care in patients with acute abdominal pain? *BMJ* 1991; **302**: 1495–1497.

12. Ohmann C, Yang Q, Franke K. Diagnostic scores for acute appendicitis. Abdominal Pain Study Group. *Eur J Surg* 1995; **161**: 273–281.

13. Rao PM, Rhea JT, Rao JA *et al*. Plain abdominal radiography in clinically suspected appendicitis: diagnostic yield, resource use, and comparison with CT. *Am J Emerg Med* 1999; **17**: 325–328.

14. Puylaert JB, Rutgers PH, Lalisang RI *et al*. A prospective study of ultrasonography in the diagnosis of appendicitis. *N Engl J Med* 1987; **317**: 666–669.

15. Allemann F, Cassina P, Rothlin M *et al*. Ultrasound scans done by surgeons for patients with acute abdominal pain: a prospective study. *Eur J Surg* 1999; **165**: 966–970.

16. Orr RK, Porter D, Hartman D. Ultrasonography to evaluate adults for appendicitis: decision making based on meta-analysis and probabilistic reasoning. *Acad Emerg Med* 1995; **2**: 644–650.

17. Rao PM, Rhea JT, Novelline RA *et al*. Effect of computed tomography of the appendix on treatment of patients and use of hospital resources. *N Engl J Med* 1998; **338**: 141–146.

18. Wise SW, Labuski MR, Kasales CJ *et al*. Comparative assessment of CT and sonographic techniques for appendiceal imaging. *AJR Am J Roentgenol* 2001; **176**: 933–941.

19. Poortman P, Lohle PN, Schoemaker CM *et al*. Comparison of CT and sonography in the diagnosis of acute appendicitis: a blinded prospective study. *AJR Am J Roentgenol* 2003; **181**: 1355–1359.

20. Van den Broek WT, Bijnen AB, van Eerten PV *et al*. Selective use of diagnostic laparoscopy in patients with suspected appendicitis. *Surg Endosc* 2000; **14**: 938–941.

21. Borgstein PJ, Cuesta MA. Acute appendicitis. A clear-cut case in men and a guessing game in women. A prospective role for diagnostic laparoscopy. *Surg Endosc* 1997; **11**: 923–927.

22. Sauerland S, Lefering R, Neugebauer EAM. Laparoscopic versus open surgery for suspected appendicitis. *Cochrane Database Syst Rev* 2007; (4) CD001546.

23. Cuesta MA, Eijsbouts QAJ, Gordijn RV *et al*. Diagnostic laparoscopy in patients with an acute abdomen of uncertain etiology. *Surg Endosc* 1998; **12**: 915–917.

24. Lau WY, Leung KL, Kwong KH *et al*. A randomized study comparing laparoscopic versus open repair of perforated peptic ulcer using suture or sutureless technique. *Ann Surg* 1996; **224**: 131–138.

25. Siu WT, Leong HT, Law BK *et al*. Laparoscopic repair for perforated peptic ulcer: a randomized controlled trial. *Ann Surg* 2002; **235**: 320–321.

26. Lau H. Laparoscopic repair of perforated peptic ulcer: a meta-analysis. *Surg Endosc* 2004; **18**: 1013–1021.

27. Lunevicius R, Morkevicius M. Systematic review comparing laparoscopic and open repair for perforated peptic ulcer. *Surg Endosc* 2005; **19**: 1565–1571.

28. Sanabria AE, Morales CH, Villegas MI. Laparoscopic repair for perforated peptic ulcer

disease. Cochrane Database Syst Rev. 2005; (4) CD004778.

29. Hinchey EJ, Schaal PG, Richards GK. Treatment of perforated diverticular disease of the colon. *Adv Surg* 1978; **12**: 85–109.

30. O'Sullivan GC, Murphy D, O'Brien MG **et al**. Laparoscopic management of generalized peritonitis due to perforated colonic diverticula. *Am J Surg* 1996; **171**: 432–434.

31. Myers E, Hurley M, O'Sullivan GC *et al*. Laparoscopic peritoneal lavage for generalized peritonitis due to perforated diverticulitis. *Br J Surg* 2008; **95**: 97–101.

32. Targarona E, Balague C. Stenting of obstructing colonic cancer: a real advance or an irrelevance to the laparoscopic surgeon ? *Surg Endosc* 2005; **19**: 745–746.

33. Trickland P, Lourie DJ, Suddelson EA, Blitz JB, Stain SC. Is laparoscopy safe and effective for treatment of acute small-bowel obstruction? *Surg Endosc* 1999; **13**: 695–698.

34. Sauerland S, Agresta F, Bergamaschi R *et al*. Laparoscopy for abdominal emergencies: evidence-based guidelines of the European Association for Endoscopic Surgery. *Surg Endosc* 2006; **20**: 14–29.

35. Ghosheh B, Salameh JR. Laparoscopic approach to acute small bowel obstruction: review of 1061 cases. *Surg Endosc* 2007; **21**: 1945–1949.

36. Levard H, Boudet MJ, Msika S *et al*. Laparoscopic treatment of acute small bowel obstruction: a multicentre retrospective study. *Aust NZ J Surg* 2001; **71**: 641–646.

Gabriel C. Oniscu John A.C. Buckels

4

General surgical procedures after liver or kidney transplantation

There have been remarkable improvements in the results of both renal and liver transplantation in the last decade: median survival of a renal graft now exceeds 12 years and that for a liver exceeds 20 years. Thus, with the increase in the post-transplant population, it is increasingly common for general surgeons, without experience in transplantation, to encounter these patients either electively in out-patient surgical clinics or presenting as an emergency with problems unrelated to the transplant procedure.

The management of transplant recipients requiring elective or emergency general surgical procedure is often complex. Not only is significant surgical expertise required to limit complications, but operating on such patients carries the additional risks due to the side effects of the immunosuppression (sepsis, renal impairment, reduced wound healing). A multidisciplinary team approach is essential and input from the transplant team (both transplant surgeons and physicians) is mandatory to ensure a successful outcome. This is particularly important in the context of an emergency presentation when lack of experience in the management of complex patients could have significant unintended long-term consequences.

This chapter summarises the main management issues in liver or kidney transplant recipients in the context of elective or emergency surgical procedures.

PRINCIPLES OF MANAGEMENT

The main complicating factor for all liver and renal transplant recipients undergoing interval surgical procedures is that they are receiving life-long

Gabriel C. Oniscu MD FRCS
Specialist Registrar, Liver Unit, Queen Elizabeth Hospital, Edgbaston, Birmingham B15 2TH, UK
E-mail: Gabriel.Oniscu@uhb.nhs.uk

John A.C. Buckels CBE MD FRCS (for correspondence)
Professor of Hepatobiliary & Transplant Surgery, Liver Unit, Queen Elizabeth Hospital, Edgbaston, Birmingham B15 2TH, UK. E-mail: John.Buckels@uhb.nhs.uk

Table 1 Immunosuppressive medications and their main side-effects

Medication	Side effects
Tacrolimus	Nephrotoxicity Diabetes Hypertension Neurotoxicity
Cyclosporin	Nephrotoxicity Gingival hypertrophy Hirsutism Hypertension
Azathioprine	Pancytopenia Pancreatitis
Mycophenolate mofetil (MMF)	Diarrhoea Pancytopenia
Prednisolone	Impaired wound healing Diabetes Peptic ulcer disease Pancreatitis
Sirolimus/Everolimus	Impaired wound healing Pancytopenia Hyper-triglyceridaemia

immunosuppressive medication. The most widely used combinations are tacrolimus or cyclosporin in combination with azathioprine or mycophenolate mofetil and steroids. Increasing numbers of patients will have had induction therapy at the time of their transplant and smaller numbers of patients receive sirolimus/everolimus. The immunosuppressive regimens vary depending on the type of transplant, the perceived risk of rejection for a particular patient and the time after transplantation. In general, with increasing time from transplantation there is a reduction in the amount of immunosuppressive medication a patient receives. These drugs have significant side effects which place the patient in a high-risk group for any surgical procedure (Table 1). It is also important to be aware that some of these agents could be responsible for the emergency presentation of the patient, as a consequence of their side-effect profile. Moreover, immunosuppressive drugs, particularly steroids, can diminish the stress response, masking physical signs in acute abdominal emergency conditions.[1]

PRE-OPERATIVE MANAGEMENT

The pre-operative evaluation of transplant recipients undergoing general surgical procedures has two distinct components. First, the diagnosis and investigation of the presenting condition, with adequate resuscitation in case of emergency presentation, should be the main aim of management. This should follow the same protocols as for any other patient presenting with that particular condition. Second, attention to the immunosuppressive regimen and the impact of the presenting disease on the function of the transplanted organ is an equally important aspect. Ideally, this latter aspect should be managed with input from the transplant team.

During the pre-operative work-up, the immunosuppressive medication should be administered as scheduled and any changes in the dosing or route of administration, which may be required in the case of sepsis or organ dysfunction, should be directed by the transplant team. Special attention to renal function is required, particularly in patients presenting with acute surgical conditions and sepsis. If a patient already has pre-existing transplant dysfunction, additional investigations and measures to optimise the function of the transplanted organ before surgery may be required. Pre-operative optimisation after close liaison with the transplant team is essential for emergency cases as these patients have a significantly higher risk of complications and organ dysfunction.

Key points 1 & 2

- Use routine laboratory tests to assess baseline function of the transplanted organ (urea and electrolytes, liver function tests and clotting studies such as international normalised ratio [INR]).

- Discuss peri-operative immunosuppressive medication with the transplant team.

INTRA-OPERATIVE MANAGEMENT

Careful surgical and anaesthetic techniques, with good communication between the surgeon and the anaesthetist, with minimal blood loss and no haemodynamic instability are the key to a smooth postoperative course. The anaesthetic team should be aware of the risks for immunosuppressed patients, particularly they should avoid potential drug interactions. In patients with good transplant function, there is no need for a change in the anaesthetic technique or drugs. However, in patients with impaired liver transplant function, hepatotoxic drugs should be avoided and the dose of drugs requiring acetylation should be reduced, as this process is diminished in poorly functioning grafts.[2] Similarly, in renal transplant recipients with impaired function or liver transplant patients with renal dysfunction, the dose of drugs requiring renal metabolism should be reduced according to the estimated renal function. The estimated glomerular filtration rate (e-GFR) is a good indicator of the renal function without performing additional invasive renal function measurements.

POSTOPERATIVE MANAGEMENT

After surgery, the principles of management for the presenting condition should be followed. From a transplant point of view, management should focus on the immunosuppressive medication and renal function. The immunosuppressive medication can usually be continued as scheduled and, whenever possible, should be administered orally (intestinal absorption is usually adequate even in the presence of postoperative ileus).[3] There are significant risks in using the intravenous forms of the calcineurin inhibitors (cyclosporin and tacrolimus) and these should not be utilised without clear guidance from the transplant team. Acute rejection due to a brief reduction in immunosuppression is uncommon and most patients will tolerate missing a limited number of doses of their normal regimens without mishap. However, if a patient requires a temporary switch to intravenous administration, this should be done after seeking advice from the transplant team. The team should also be contacted if unexpected complications arise, such as sepsis or deteriorating renal function, which are likely to require a reduction in the maintenance doses. The long-term use of steroids in transplant recipients has raised concerns regarding the risk of peri-operative adrenocortical insufficiency. In general, this risk is minimal and patients seldom need additional steroids, but can be maintained on their pre-procedure dose.[1,3]

Tacrolimus and cyclosporin are metabolised through the cytochrome P450 microsomal enzyme pathway; therefore, one should be aware of those drugs that interfere with this pathway and could lead to either toxic levels (erythromycin, clarithromycin, fluconazole, nifedipine, diltiazem) or decreased levels of immunosuppression (rifampicin, phenitoin). In the peri-operative period, trough levels should be measured daily until the patient is stable, any ileus has resolved and there is good oral intake.

In patients with impaired renal function, drug administration should be tailored to the level of renal function. Pain control should be readily achieved by a combination of paracetamol, tramadol, morphine and the use of patient-controlled analgesia (PCA) or epidural. Non-steroidal anti-inflammatory drugs should be avoided due to their potentially nephrotoxic effects which can be additive to that of the baseline immunosuppression and could lead to severe renal dysfunction.

Hypertension is common in transplant patients. If the patient is already on anti-hypertensive medication, this can often be omitted during the peri-operative period (epidural analgesia, if utilised, often has a lowering effect on blood pressure) but will need restarting within a few days. New medication may be required in some patients though this should be done with the advice of the transplant team noting that certain drugs such as doxazosin should be avoided due to the interaction with the cytochrome P450 pathway.

Impaired wound healing is a potential problem for surgical procedures in immunosuppressed patients especially in those receiving sirolimus or everolimus (inhibitors of TOR – 'target of rapamycin' – a key regulatory kinase in the process of cell division).[4] These drugs are finding favour in the longer term management of transplant recipients as they do not exhibit the nephrotoxicity seen with the calcineurin inhibitor drugs. They impair wound healing via a mechanism involving the inhibition of smooth muscle cell proliferation and reduced collagen deposition. Experimental data have shown diminished expression of VEGF and nitric oxide in wounds[5] and with intestinal anastomoses.[6] The concomitant use of steroids and sirolimus has a synergistic effect[7] and this combination of immunosuppressive agents is usually avoided in the immediate post-transplant period. However, most general surgical procedures in transplant recipients take place beyond 3 months after transplantation when some patients may be receiving sirolimus or everolimus. The benefit of maintaining the patient on these agents versus the risk of wound-healing problems should be assessed by the transplant team who will base the decision to switch to other drugs on the graft function and the presence of associated risk factors such as diabetes and obesity.

> ### Key point 3
>
> - Follow the principles of management for the presenting condition but avoid non-steroidal analgesics.

GENERAL SURGICAL PROCEDURES

Some of the general surgical procedures in liver or renal transplant recipients are related to complications of transplantation (such as biliary strictures or ureteric strictures) and should only be managed by the transplant team. Sometimes, their presentation cannot be differentiated from that of unrelated surgical conditions and, if the patient presents to the local surgical team, after an initial evaluation and resuscitation, early referral back to the transplant team is mandatory.

> ### Key points 4 & 5
>
> - All major general surgical interventions should be discussed with the transplant team or should be carried out under joint care.
>
> - All transplant-related complications should be managed by the transplant teams.

MINOR PROCEDURES

Minor surgical procedures such as excision of skin lesions, small lumps or incision and drainage of abscesses do not require an extensive pre-operative work-up and could be carried out as day-cases. The function of the transplanted organ should be documented with particular attention to the coagulation tests. The risk of infection or wound healing problems is small (1.5–3%) if the steroids dose is less than 15 mg/day,[3] but increases significantly with higher doses. Therefore, unless there is a diagnostic urgency, these procedures should be performed when the steroids dose is below this level. There are no specific reports of impaired wound healing for patients on sirolimus undergoing minor surgery. It should be noted that all skin lesions removed from immunosuppressed patients should be submitted to histology due to the high risk of cutaneous malignancy in these patients.

> ### Key point 6
>
> - Minor surgical procedures can be safely performed by general surgical teams.

CHOLELITHIASIS AND KIDNEY TRANSPLANTATION

The management of gallstone disease in patients awaiting renal transplantation has been controversial. Recent guidelines suggest that patients with symptomatic gallstones should undergo laparoscopic cholecystectomy to prevent further complications and the increased morbidity associated with immunosuppressive medication if surgery was deferred until after transplantation. The incidence of asymptomatic gallstone disease in the transplant population matches that in the general population with similar risks of acute cholecystitis.[8] Although early reports[9] suggested an increased risk of later serious complications with conservative management, recent studies found no increased morbidity related to asymptomatic cholelithiasis or other gallbladder pathologies after kidney transplantation.[10] Asymptomatic gallstone disease should be managed conservatively. Surgery is indicated when patients become symptomatic.[11]

HERNIA REPAIR

Immunosuppression can delay wound healing and predisposes to a higher incidence of incisional hernias. In the case of liver transplantation, the degree of malnutrition, the amount of ascites, the length of intensive care unit (ICU) stay,[12] re-intervention for postoperative complications,[13] and a combined transverse and midline incision[14] are additional risk factors for the development of incisional hernias. The reported incidence of incisional hernia after liver transplantation varies between 5%[15] and 17%[14] whilst the risk of incisional hernia after kidney transplantation is much lower (1% and 4%).[16] In general, incisional hernias develop early after transplant but can occur late. Presentation is usually with abdominal discomfort and only 5% present with obstruction.[13]

There is debate surrounding the optimal surgical technique for incisional hernia repair in transplant recipients, particularly regarding the use of polypropylene mesh. Mesh infection in immunosuppressed patients can have disastrous consequences; therefore, this risk has to be balanced against the lower risk of hernia recurrence. Recent data suggest that recurrence rates following mesh repair are significantly lower compared to primary repair (9% versus 20%)[17,18] and are not associated with higher complication rates.[12] Consequently, mesh repair (sublay, onlay or even inlay)[12,19] is increasingly used in the management of incisional hernias following renal[19] as well as liver[12,14] transplantation. Given the proximity of the hernia to the transplanted organ, it is recommended that these procedures should usually be carried out by the transplant team.

Inguinal hernias can be repaired respecting the same principles as in non-transplant patients, mesh repair being the preferred technique in most centres. Umbilical hernias are more common in liver recipients (often related to pretransplant ascites), can be repaired using conventional techniques and do not normally require the use of mesh.

ELECTIVE COLONIC SURGERY

Elective colonic surgery is relatively uncommon in renal transplant recipients, unless the patients develop colonic malignancy as a consequence of long-term immunosuppression. In these cases, the management should respect the principles outlined earlier and should be carried out by colorectal surgeons in close co-operation with the transplant team. Most colonic complications following renal transplantation occur in an emergency setting and will be discussed below.

Elective colonic surgery following liver transplantation is more common due to the association of inflammatory bowel disease (IBD) with primary sclerosing cholangitis for which transplantation may be required. Many of the medications used after liver transplantation have been used to treat IBD. Despite an expectation that patients at risk should have a milder course due to the immunosuppressive agents, symptomatic IBD can be a significant problem necessitating aggressive medical therapy and, sometimes, surgery. Furthermore, *de novo* IBD has been reported in patients transplanted for primary sclerosing cholangitis (PSC) or auto-immune hepatitis.[20] In these patients, the presence of cytomegalovirus mismatch (positive donor to negative recipient) as well as the use of tacrolimus were significant risk factors for the development of the disease.

Patients with IBD who have not undergone a colectomy prior to liver transplantation should be managed collaboratively by both the transplant hepatologists and the gastroenterologists. Regular surveillance is essential, given the risk of colon cancer developing in patients with ulcerative colitis after liver transplantation. The highest risk is in those with pancolitis or dysplasia on a background of more than a 10-year history of colitis.[21,22] Colectomy is advocated in the high-risk cases and in those that do not respond to best medical therapy.[23] The timing of surgery is important. It has been shown that colectomy is a relatively safe procedure when associated with a liver transplant for PSC; therefore, it should be considered prior to, or shortly after, the transplant in selected patients.[22]

Key point 7

- Elective colorectal surgery should only be performed in colorectal units that work closely with liver transplant units and not under-taken by surgeons unfamiliar with the management of transplant patients.

EMERGENCY SURGERY

Emergency surgery in transplant recipients carries a higher risk of compli-cations compared to elective cases. Furthermore, the immunosuppression contributes to the risks and may also mask the presentation leading to a delay in diagnosis. Therefore, these cases are best managed in conjunction with the transplant units if the time allows for a safe transfer, or after seeking advice from the unit prior to embarking on the emergency treatment of the condition.

Upper GI emergencies
Immunosuppression carries an increased risk of upper GI complications and, in particular, peptic ulcer disease with perforation and bleeding. Steroids

particularly high-dose steroids used to treat acute rejection episodes are associated with the highest risk of perforated peptic disease. This has now almost disappeared, with the advent of proton pump inhibitor drugs which are usually given to all patients taking steroids. If a perforation occurs, the same principles of management as for non-transplant patients should be followed. In the case of liver graft recipients, surgery is technically more challenging due to upper abdominal adhesions and the involvement of the transplant surgeon in any procedures is recommended if practicable.

Appendicitis

While appendicitis is one of the most common surgical emergencies, with an estimated life-time risk of 6–8%, there are very few reports of the condition in renal or liver transplant recipients. The reported incidence varies between 0.2% and 1.81%[24] and most patients present with classical symptoms (right iliac fossa pain, nausea, vomiting) but not necessarily leukocytosis.[25] The diagnosis is essentially clinical but occasionally computed tomography can help when there has been a delay in presentation.[24] Treatment should follow the same principles as for non-transplant patients, but patients should be made aware of a higher complication rate and longer hospital stay.

Colonic surgery

Most of the data about colonic emergencies in transplant recipients comes from renal transplantation. Colonic complications include perforation, ischaemic colitis, ulceration and enterocolitis. The overall incidence of these complications is low at around 2% but carries high mortality with reported rates ranging between 16% and 70%.[26–29] Overall, perforation is the most common complication and is associated with pre-existing pathology such as diverticular disease in the majority of cases.[30] Physical signs can often be masked by immunosuppression. The incidence of perforations seems to be associated with the higher level of immunosuppression in the first 3 months after transplant,[29] although late cases have also been reported.

Once a diagnosis is made, colonic perforations require immediate treatment which consists of adequate resuscitation, antibiotic therapy, reduction of the doses of immunosuppressive medication and timely surgery. It is generally agreed that resection of the perforated segment with exteriorisation of the bowel ends is a safer option than primary anastomosis, which should be reserved for right colonic perforations[31] or left-sided perforations with minimal peritoneal contamination.[32]

Colonic ulceration with subsequent perforation has been described with cytomegalovirus,[33] varicella virus, *Candida* spp., actinomyces or severe MRSA infection.[34] Patients will present with colonic haemorrhage and diarrhoea and usually deteriorating renal function. Despite surgical treatment, these conditions are associated with a high mortality rate. There is limited data about *Clostridium difficile* colitis in renal transplant recipients but there are indications that around 5% of patients require emergency colectomy for toxic megacolon following the initial clostridial infection.[35]

Faecal impaction after renal transplantation can affect the right colon and present as small bowel obstruction or chronic constipation. The causes are unknown, but inhibition of vagal motor activity secondary to uraemia, immunosuppressive medication and antihypertensive medication have been proposed.[28] The risk is increased by postoperative ileus, dehydration and bed rest.[36] With adequate management, the risk of perforation should be minimal.

Ischaemic colitis is rare in liver transplant recipients but has been described in most series following renal transplantation. A number of factors may predispose to this condition: advanced atheromatous disease (a hallmark of long-term dialysis patients), heart failure, retroperitoneal dissection, peri-operative hypotension and immunosuppressive medication.[28] Surgery is usually futile and surviving cases are anecdotal.

Acute colonic pseudo-obstruction (Ogilvie's syndrome) is a rare complication following liver or renal transplantation. Association with steroid therapy or cytomegalovirus infection (with remission following anti-viral treatment)[37,38] has been described. Colonoscopic decompression is successful in 87–97% of cases[39–41] and should be associated with reduction in steroid doses in cases where a definite causal relationship has been identified. Delayed diagnosis with bowel necrosis and perforation carries a very high mortality.[42]

Key point 8

- Emergency colorectal surgery in transplant recipients is associated with a high mortality and cases are best dealt with by the transplant surgical team jointly with the colorectal team.

CONCLUSIONS

With the increasing number of long-term survivors following liver and kidney transplantation, the general surgeon will increasingly encounter these patients on an elective or emergency basis. Their management can be complex and challenging and it should not be undertaken lightly. Even in experienced hands, elective general surgical procedures in transplant recipients are associated with 15–25% morbidity, which is higher in an emergency setting. Therefore, the decision to embark upon surgical procedures should be based on experience and the availability of advice from the transplant team.

Minor procedures do not require changes to the transplant management and have negligible impact on the function of the transplanted organ. These cases could be managed locally where appropriate surgical expertise and transplant advice is readily available. However, much of the elective and emergency procedures discussed above require significant input from the transplant team and should be referred back to the transplanting centre whenever possible. Involvement of other specialist teams such as colorectal ones is vital to ensure the optimal expertise in managing the presenting condition as well as the function of the transplanted organ. If these guidelines are respected, surgical procedures in transplant recipients can be carried out safely with a minimal risk of complications.

Key points for clinical practice

- Use routine laboratory tests to assess baseline function of the transplanted organ (urea and electrolytes, liver function tests and clotting studies such as international normalised ratio [INR]).

- Discuss peri-operative immunosuppressive medication with the transplant team.

- Follow the principles of management for the presenting condition but avoid non-steroidal analgesics.

- All major general surgical interventions should be discussed with the transplant team or should be carried out under joint care.

- All transplant-related complications should be managed by the transplant teams.

- Minor surgical procedures can be safely performed by general surgical teams.

- Elective colorectal surgery should only be performed in colorectal units that work closely with liver transplant units and not undertaken by surgeons unfamiliar with the management of transplant patients.

- Emergency colorectal surgery in transplant recipients is associated with a high mortality and cases are best dealt with by the transplant surgical team jointly with the colorectal team.

References

1. Bromberg JS, Baliga P, Cofer JB, Rajagopalan PR, Friedman RJ. Stress steroids are not required for patients receiving a renal allograft and undergoing operation. *J Am Coll Surg* 1995; **180**: 532–536.
2. Baubillier EDP. Anaesthetic management of patients with alcoholic liver disease. *Baillières Clin Anaesthesiol* 1992; **6**: 847–859.
3. Testa G, Goldstein RM, Toughanipour A *et al*. Guidelines for surgical procedures after liver transplantation. *Ann Surg* 1998; **227**: 590–599.
4. Dean PG. Wound-healing complications after kidney transplantation: a prospective, randomized comparison of sirolimus and tacrolimus. *Transplantation* 2004; **77**: 1555–1561.
5. Schaffer MSR. Sirolimus impairs wound healing. *Langenbecks Arch Surg* 2007; **392**: 297–303.
6. van der Vliet JAWM. Everolimus interferes with healing of experimental intestinal anastomoses. *Transplantation* 2006; **82**: 1477–1483.
7. Gaber MWAA. Changes in abdominal wounds following treatment with sirolimus and steroids in a rat model. *Transplant Proc* 2006; **38**: 3331–3332.
8. Greenstein SM, Katz S, Sun S *et al*. Prevalence of asymptomatic cholelithiasis and risk of acute cholecystitis after kidney transplantation. *Transplantation* 1997; **63**: 1030–1032.
9. Graham SM, Flowers JL, Schweitzer E, Bartlett ST, Imbembo AL. The utility of prophylactic laparoscopic cholecystectomy in transplant candidates. *Am J Surg* 1995; **169**: 44–48.
10. Jackson T, Treleaven D, Arlen D, D'Sa A, Lambert K, Birch DW. Management of asymptomatic cholelithiasis for patients awaiting renal transplantation. *Surg Endosc* 2005; **19**: 510–513.
11. Kao LS, Flowers C, Flum DR. Prophylactic cholecystectomy in transplant patients: a decision analysis. *J Gastrointest Surg* 2005; **9**: 965–972.

12. Muller V, Lehner M, Klein P, Hohenberger W, Ott R. Incisional hernia repair after orthotopic liver transplantation: a technique employing an inlay/onlay polypropylene mesh. *Langenbecks Arch Surg* 2003; **388**: 167–173.

13. Vardanian AJ, Farmer DG, Ghobrial RM, Busuttil RW, Hiatt JR. Incisional hernia after liver transplantation. *J Am Coll Surg* 2006; **203**: 421–425.

14. Janssen H, Lange R, Erhard J, Malago M, Eigler FW, Broelsch CE. Causative factors, surgical treatment and outcome of incisional hernia after liver transplantation. *Br J Surg* 2002; **89**: 1049–1054.

15. Piazzese E, Montalti R, Beltempo P et al. Incidence, predisposing factors, and results of surgical treatment of incisional hernia after orthotopic liver transplantation. *Transplant Proc* 2004; **36**: 3097–3098.

16. Mazzucchi E, Nahas WC, Antonopoulos I, Ianhez LE, Arap S. Incisional hernia and its repair with polypropylene mesh in renal transplant recipients. *J Urol* 2001; **166**: 816–819.

17. Antonopoulos IM, Nahas WC, Mazzucchi E, Piovesan AC, Birolini C, Lucon AM. Is polypropylene mesh safe and effective for repairing infected incisional hernia in renal transplant recipients? *Urology* 2005; **66**: 874–877.

18. Li EN, Silverman RP, Goldberg NH. Incisional hernia repair in renal transplantation patients. *Hernia* 2005; **9**: 231–237.

19. Birolini C, Mazzucchi E, Utiyama EM et al. Prosthetic repair of incisional hernia in kidney transplant patients. A technique with onlay polypropylene mesh. *Hernia* 2001; **5**: 31–35.

20. Verdonk RC, Dijkstra G, Haagsma EB et al. Inflammatory bowel disease after liver transplantation: risk factors for recurrence and *de novo* disease. *Am J Transplant* 2006; **6**: 1422–1429.

21. Bleday R, Lee E, Jessurun J, Heine J, Wong WD. Increased risk of early colorectal neoplasms after hepatic transplant in patients with inflammatory bowel disease. *Dis Colon Rectum* 1993; **36**: 908–912.

22. Vera A, Gunson BK, Ussatoff V et al. Colorectal cancer in patients with inflammatory bowel disease after liver transplantation for primary sclerosing cholangitis. *Transplantation* 2003; **75**: 1983–1988.

23. Befeler AS, Lissoos TW, Schiano TD et al. Clinical course and management of inflammatory bowel disease after liver transplantation. *Transplantation* 1998; **65**: 393–396.

24. Savar A, Hiatt JR, Busuttil RW. Acute appendicitis after solid organ transplantation. *Clin Transplant* 2006; **20**: 78–80.

25. Abt PL, Abdullah I, Korenda K et al. Appendicitis among liver transplant recipients. *Liver Transpl* 2005; **11**: 1282–1284.

26. Ressetta G, Simeth C, Ziza F, La Bruna D, Balani A. [Colonic diverticulosis complicated with perforation. Analysis of several prognosis variables and criteria for emergency surgery]. *Ann Ital Chir* 1998; **69**: 63–70.

27. McCune TR, Nylander WA, Van Buren DH et al. Colonic screening prior to renal transplantation and its impact on post-transplant colonic complications. *Clin Transplant* 1992; **6**: 91–96.

28. Archibald SD, Jirsch DW, Bear RA. Gastrointestinal complications of renal transplantation. 2. The colon. *Can Med Assoc J* 1978; **119**: 1301–1305, 1309.

29. Stelzner M, Vlahakos DV, Milford EL, Tilney NL. Colonic perforations after renal transplantation. *J Am Coll Surg* 1997; **184**: 63–69.

30. Soravia C, Baldi A, Kartheuser A et al. Acute colonic complications after kidney transplantation. *Acta Chir Belg* 1995; **95**: 157–161.

31. Isbister WH. The management of colorectal perforation and peritonitis. *Aust NZ J Surg* 1997; **67**: 804–808.

32. Seiler CA, Brugger L, Maurer CA, Renzulli P, Buchler MW. [Peritonitis in diverticulitis: the Bern concept]. *Zentralbl Chir* 1998; **123**: 1394–1399.

33. Toogood GJ, Gillespie PH, Gujral S et al. Cytomegalovirus infection and colonic perforation in renal transplant patients. *Transpl Int* 1996; **9**: 248–251.

34. Nomura T, Tasaki Y, Hirata Y et al. Intestinal perforation after cadaveric renal transplantation. *Int J Urol* 2004; **11**: 774–777.

35. Keven K, Basu A, Re L et al. *Clostridium difficile* colitis in patients after kidney and pancreas-kidney transplantation. *Transpl Infect Dis* 2004; **6**: 10–14.

36. Aguilo JJ, Zincke H, Woods JE, Buckingham JM. Intestinal perforation due to fecal impaction after renal transplantation. *J Urol* 1976; **116**: 153–155.

37. Shapiro AM, Bain VG, Preiksaitis JK, Ma MM, Issa S, Kneteman NM. Ogilvie's syndrome associated with acute cytomegaloviral infection after liver transplantation. *Transpl Int* 2000; **13**: 41–45.

38. Shrestha BM, Darby C, Fergusson C, Lord R, Salaman JR, Moore RH. Cytomegalovirus causing acute colonic pseudo-obstruction in a renal transplant recipient. *Postgrad Med J* 1996; **72**: 429–430.

39. Stratta RJ, Starling JR, D'Alessandro AM *et al.* Acute colonic ileus (pseudo-obstruction) in renal transplant recipients. *Surgery* 1988; **104**: 616–623.

40. Koneru B, Selby R, O'Hair DP, Tzakis AG, Hakala TR, Starzl TE. Nonobstructing colonic dilatation and colon perforations following renal transplantation. *Arch Surg* 1990; **125**: 610–613.

41. O'Malley KJ, Flechner SM, Kapoor A *et al.* Acute colonic pseudo-obstruction (Ogilvie's syndrome) after renal transplantation. *Am J Surg* 1999; **177**: 492–496.

42. Pokorny H, Plochl W, Soliman T *et al.* Acute colonic pseudo-obstruction (Ogilvie's-syndrome) and pneumatosis intestinalis in a kidney recipient patient. *Wien Klin Wochenschr* 2003; **115**: 732–735.

Samer Humadi Richard Welbourn

5

Bariatric surgery: rationale, development and current status

Obesity is a chronic, relapsing, debilitating, life-long disease, officially recognised by the World Health Organization (WHO) as a global pandemic.[1] There is now more obesity than malnutrition and the future cost of healthcare for the obese threatens to overwhelm available resources. Bariatric surgery is the only effective means of achieving long-term weight loss in the severely obese, but is only used in less than 1% of those eligible for it. A burgeoning medical and surgical literature supports its rapid adoption.[2,3] The international guidelines on patient suitability for surgery are a body mass index (BMI) $> 40 \, \text{kg/m}^2$ or BMI $> 35 \, \text{kg/m}^2$ together with obesity-related disease (National Institutes of Health, 1991).[4]

Obesity, defined as a BMI of $30 \, \text{kg/m}^2$ or more, affects 1.7 billion people world-wide. The epidemic is worst in the US, where more than 30% of adults are obese.[3] The main reasons appear to be a combination of less active life-styles and changes in eating patterns.[2] The adult epidemic is paralleled by a childhood epidemic; because of this, it seems certain that the global prevalence will continue to rise for the foreseeable future.

Severe obesity is associated with harmful co-morbidity, including type 2 diabetes mellitus, hypertension, dyslipidaemia, obstructive sleep apnoea, polycystic ovarian syndrome, non-alcoholic steatohepatosis, asthma, back and lower limb degenerative problems, cancer and depression.[4] These cause more than 2.5 million premature deaths per year world-wide.[5] Obesity costs the National Health Service £500 million per year and the UK as a whole £7.4 billion

Samer Humadi FRCS
Specialist Registrar, Department of Upper Gastrointestinal and Bariatric Surgery, Musgrove Park Hospital, Taunton, Somerset TA1 5DA, UK. samer1996@hotmail.com

Richard Welbourn MD FRCS (for correspondence)
Cosultant Gastrointestinal Surgeon, Department of Upper Gastrointestinal and Bariatric Surgery, Musgrove Park Hospital, Taunton, Somerset TA1 5DA, UK
E-mail: richard.welbourn@tst.nhs.uk

per year.[6] In the US, healthcare costs of obesity are estimated at \$92.6 billion per year. The treatment of morbid obesity and its co-morbidities thus places a huge burden on healthcare providers.

Traditional approaches to weight loss including diet, exercise and medication achieve no more than 5–10% reduction in body weight, with high recidivism rates.[2,7] Bariatric surgery (from the Greek meaning 'the medicine and surgery of weight') achieves sustained, long-term weight loss durable to at least 15 years[8] and causes remarkable improvements in co-morbidity.[3] As a result, it is fast becoming the quickest developing area of surgery in the US and Europe. In 2002, about 55,000 obesity operations were performed in the US and in 2006 there were 200,000,[9] a total that now exceeds the number of cholecystectomies. The UK lags far behind the rest of the world in bariatric surgery, with only 347 publicly funded operations in 2004 for a population of nearly 50 million.[10]

Key point 1

- Bariatric surgery is the only effective long-term treatment for severe obesity.

AIMS OF BARIATRIC SURGERY

Bariatric surgery aims to reduce the excess mortality and morbidity of obesity. Percentage excess weight loss or BMI change is taken as the main measure of success using 25 kg/m^2 as the notional ideal BMI, with success generally defined as > 50% excess weight loss or BMI < 35 kg/m^2.[11] Measurement of co-morbidity is often necessarily qualitative with outcomes usually reported as resolved, improved, the same or worse. Reduced medication usage is a relatively quantitative end-point and is taken to indicate improvement in co-morbid disease.[3] Patient-reported end-points include quality-of-life scores using instruments such as the Bariatric Analysis and Reporting Outcome System (BAROS).[12]

PATIENT ASSESSMENT FOR SURGERY

There is strong agreement on the need for a comprehensive multidisciplinary process that includes patient education about the available procedures. The team should include dedicated surgeons, physicians, nutritionists, nurses and patient support.[13,14] Endocrine causes, although rare, must be excluded and co-morbidity must be ameliorated so that operative risk is minimised. Few data are available on operative risk assessment and there is an urgent need to establish risk scores so that outcomes can be compared between centres.[15,16] Patients and clinical teams must be committed to long-term follow-up;[2] in fact, the Surgical Review Corporation of the American Society for Metabolic and Bariatric Surgery (ASMBS) mandates 75% 5-year follow-up rates before designation as a 'Center of Excellence'.[17] The team approach characteristic of high-volume hospitals appears to facilitate better outcomes.[13]

Key point 2

- Education and multidisciplinary assessment are essential to optimise patient preparation for surgery; commitment by the team and patient to long-term follow-up is mandatory.

SURGICAL PROCEDURES FOR OBESITY

The development of surgical procedures for obesity has been reviewed by Deitel and Shikora.[18] In the 1950s, the jejunocolic bypass was developed after it was noted that individuals who had the short-bowel syndrome lost weight. In the 1960s and early 1970s, this evolved into the jejuno-ileal bypass. However, this operation led to severe metabolic complications including malnutrition, renal and liver dysfunction, osteomalacia and osteoporosis due to the blind loop produced and it quickly became obsolete.

ROUX-EN-Y GASTRIC BYPASS

In the 1960s, Mason and Ito[19] initiated the gastric bypass using a jejunal loop[9] which evolved to a Roux-en-Y configuration to eliminate bile reflux. Currently, Roux-en-Y gastric bypass, followed by gastric banding, is the commonest bariatric operation world-wide. The laparoscopic approach to Roux-en-Y gastric bypass has been rapidly adopted since the landmark report in 1994 by Wittgrove et al.[20] Although it has a steep learning curve, laparoscopic Roux-en-Y gastric bypass is associated with shorter hospital stay, less pain, improved pulmonary function, and quicker improvement in quality of life compared to open Roux-en-Y gastric bypass.[21] With experience, laparoscopic Roux-en-Y gastric bypass can be performed with few complications and with early discharge.[22] Ten-year results of gastric bypass in large clinical series consistently demonstrate mean excess weight loss of 50–60%,[23–26] about 10% more than gastric banding.[27] Also, weight loss after gastric bypass is appreciably faster than with banding and may be more durable, with a lower failure rate.[27] A European matched pair analysis of laparoscopic Roux-en-Y gastric bypass and gastric banding showed better weight loss at 2 years and better improvement in type 2 diabetes mellitus and dyslipidaemia for Roux-en-Y gastric bypass.[28]

The optimal length of the jejunal Roux limb is not known. At least two randomised controlled trials have found little or no difference in weight loss between shorter or longer limbs. Malabsorption may not, therefore, be a factor in the mechanism of action, since most of the small bowel is in continuity and the operation does not lead to diarrhoea. In a non-randomised study, there was no difference at 10 years between cohorts with short or long Roux limb lengths. Currently, it is common practice for the Roux limb lengths to be made 100 cm for BMI < 50 kg/m^2 and 150 cm for BMI of 50 kg/m^2 or more.[29]

Roux-en-Y gastric bypass does lead to appreciable vitamin and micronutrient deficiency including iron and vitamin B$_{12}$, which occur in more than 30% of patients, with chronic mild anaemia being common. Patients must be committed to life-long vitamin and mineral supplements to include also calcium and folate. However, protein/calorie malnutrition after the initial catabolism during weight loss is < 1% if the Roux limb is < 150 cm.[30]

There is good evidence that at least part of the mechanism of action of Roux-en-Y gastric bypass is by changing the gut hormones that control appetite and satiety. Two of these, PYY and GLP-1, rise after surgery and are associated with loss of appetite and early satiety after eating.[31]

Key point 3

- Roux-en-Y gastric bypass is the commonest operation world-wide with 60–70% excess weight loss durable to 15 years. Access for the procedure is increasingly laparoscopic.

GASTROPLASTY

In the mid-1970s, in an effort to simplify gastric restriction, Mason *et al.*[32] developed the proximal restrictive gastroplasty. Initially, the stomach was stapled horizontally but the operation evolved to vertical stapling along the lesser curve up to the angle of His as it seemed that the thicker muscle here might be more resistant to dilatation. In addition, the outlet was banded by a mesh strip or a silastic ring to prevent enlargement.[32] Open, vertical-banded gastroplasty was widely used and has produced good weight loss, but less than following gastric bypass. However, this procedure has now been superseded by gastric banding, due to the relative ease of laparoscopic banding and its adjustability.

BILIOPANCREATIC DIVERSION

In 1976, Scopinaro *et al.*[33] performed the first biliopancreatic diversion. Leaving a biliopancreatic limb anastomosed to an alimentary limb with a comparatively short distal common limb, this operation required a partial gastrectomy to avoid marginal ulceration.[33] If the gastric remnant in the biliopancreatic diversion was too small for adequate oral intake, hypo-albuminaemia and nutritional sequelae could occur, unless a longer common limb was left. Excess weight loss from biliopancreatic diversion is 70–80%, more than for Roux-en-Y gastric bypass or gastric banding; however, after biliopancreatic diversion there is a significant risk of malnutrition, quoted at 7% long-term, and thus a high degree of nutritionist input and compliance is needed.[34]

DUODENAL SWITCH

A modification of the biliopancreatic diversion in increasing use is the 'duodenal switch'.[35] In this, the greater curve of the stomach is resected (sleeve gastrectomy, which produces gastric restriction), leaving the entire lesser curve and pylorus in continuity. By leaving the pylorus intact, dumping syndrome and marginal ulceration are prevented. The alimentary limb is anastomosed to the divided proximal duodenum (proximal to common bile duct). The biliopancreatic limb is anastomosed to the side of the alimentary limb 75–100 cm proximal to the ileocaecal valve, leaving this common limb for absorption. Excess weight loss following biliopancreatic diversion with duodenal switch is typically 80% or more; however, a concern for both procedures is diarrhoea, anaemia, calcium and protein malabsorption, and bone demineralisation. Patients require very careful long-term nutritional follow-up.

GASTRIC BANDING

In the late 1980s, adjustable gastric banding was developed, with a hollow band connected by a tube to a reservoir on the abdominal wall.[36] Fluid injection into the reservoir permits adjustment of the gastric restriction.[37] Peri-operative complications for banding are fewer than for Roux-en-Y gastric bypass, biliopancreatic diversion or duodenal switch and the peri-operative mortality is about 0.1%. However, there is a failure rate and results are highly dependent on quality of follow-up. After a high initial gastric erosion rate with a perigastric approach, it is now agreed that a pars flaccida approach, which incorporates the fatty tissue of the lesser curve within the band, should be used if possible. Band slippage is reduced by non-absorbable anterior gastro–gastric fixation sutures. Other significant problems include port-site infections, which generally necessitate band removal, and tubing problems such as disconnection and puncture from needles during attempts at reservoir fills.

A properly adjusted band that has a small 'virtual' gastric pouch above the band leads to early satiety and loss of appetite but without marked changes in gut satiety hormones. The pouch appears necessary for these sensations since a band placed entirely around the gastro-oesophageal junction produces only dysphagia and poor weight loss. Patients should be able to eat small amounts of well-chewed normal food and the band should not be too tight, otherwise patients tend to eat liquid food only.

The principal advantage of banding is its minimal invasiveness. However, long-term results are largely unknown as there are very few series with large numbers and more than 5 years' follow-up, despite the tens of thousands of bands that have been placed world-wide. A recent systematic review of weight loss following different operations at 3–10 years found few weight data at more than 5-year follow-up, and no knowledge at all of the numbers lost to follow-up.[38] The available data, however, suggest that cumulative weight loss up to 5 years in patients with bands intact is similar between standard limb Roux-en-Y gastric bypass and banding, certainly for patients starting with a lower BMI.[38] However, not included in these reports are the long-term differences in remission of co-morbidity from these two operations.

Two large European series have follow-up of more than 5 years. In one, the proportion of patients with good excess weight loss (> 50%), even in those without major complication, remained at best between 55–65%. Further, each year added 3–4% to the major complication rate, contributing significantly to the total failure rate.[39] With a success rate for banding < 50% and a failure rate approaching 40% after 7 years, these authors now perform Roux-en-Y gastric bypass as their procedure of choice. In the other series, mean excess weight loss was 59% at 8 years but there was an appreciable re-operation rate due to complications such as slippage.[40] It appears accepted that even in the best centres there is a long-term failure rate of 20% or more from gastric bands.[27]

Key point 4

- Gastric banding is a least-invasive operation with 50–60% excess weight loss over 5 years but long-term results are unknown and the complication rate may be cumulative.

OTHER PROCEDURES

Laparoscopic sleeve gastrectomy is emerging as a popular alternative to Roux-en-Y gastric bypass in higher risk patients especially those with BMI > 60 kg/m^2 since the perceived risk may be less.[41] Sleeve gastrectomy evolved from the Magenstrasse and Mill operation devised by Johnston *et al.*[42] Excess weight loss in the year after sleeve gastrectomy seems very similar to Roux-en-Y gastric bypass but there are no long-term reports yet. An advantage of this procedure is that, if there is weight re-gain later, it can be followed by other bariatric operations, *e.g.* bypass, switch or banding. Temporary placement of intragastric balloons has also gained popularity especially in Italy in an attempt to make patients fitter for surgery by initial weight loss.[43] However, they are only licensed for 6 months and weight re-gain tends to occur after removal.

EFFECTS OF BARIATRIC SURGERY ON CO-MORBIDITY

Many studies have shown that co-morbidities including diabetes and hypertension improve in the vast majority of patients at 1–2 years following Roux-en-Y gastric bypass, gastric banding and biliopancreatic diversion/duodenal switch.[3,8,27,28,33,44] In a meta-analysis of more than 22,000 patients, improvements were also found in dyslipidaemia, sleep apnoea and quality of life after bariatric surgery.[3,45] The effects on type 2 diabetes mellitus and hypertension are 'dose-related' and are greater for gastric bypass than for banding. Thus, in 1995, Pories *et al.*[46] surprisingly found that Roux-en-Y gastric bypass leads to long-term remission of type 2 diabetes (no treatment, normal HbA$_{1c}$ levels). Typically, type 2 diabetes mellitus improves within days after surgery for Roux-en-Y gastric bypass and biliopancreatic diversion/duodenal switch, long before significant weight loss has occurred. With gastric banding, improvement is proportional to weight loss and is, therefore, slower. Remission is less likely the longer type 2 diabetes mellitus has been present because of progressive β-cell deterioration over time.[44] In the meta-analysis of Buchwald *et al.*,[3] remission rates for type 2 diabetes mellitus at 2 years were 83% for Roux-en-Y gastric bypass and 47% for banding.

The mechanism of remission of type 2 diabetes mellitus is being keenly researched. Improvement in insulin resistance may be due to weight loss *per se* and production of incretins including GLP-1 (increasing insulin secretion).

Current debate focuses on changes in gut hormone secretion due to foregut bypass.[47]

Bariatric surgery, in general, is so effective at improving type 2 diabetes mellitus that, at the Diabetes Surgery Summit in Rome (March 2007), it was proposed that bariatric surgery should be considered as a treatment option for diabetics with BMI < 35 kg/m^2.[48] Although not proven, remission of diabetes is likely to halt the progression of microvascular complications.[49] It is entirely possible that further procedures specifically directed to remission of diabetes will emerge over time, such as duodenojejunal bypass.[50]

Buchwald *et al.*[3] also found that the remission rates at 2 years for high blood pressure were about 75% for Roux-en-Y gastric bypass and 38% for banding. However, the Swedish Obese Subjects study found that hypertension tended to recur over time.[8]

Key point 5

• Roux-en-Y gastric bypass, biliopancreatic diversion and duodenal switch lead to remission of diabetes in > 80% of cases, probably by hormonal mechanism as it occurs before weight loss.

WHICH OPERATION IS BEST?

The debate about which operation is best will continue for some years and other operations are likely to evolve. Choice of procedure seems to be driven by local culture, surgeon and patient preference and knowledge of risk versus benefit.[18,34,51] The popularity of banding has declined in Europe but is high in Australia. For example, in Switzerland in 1998, the ratio of banding to bypass was 20:1; however, by 2004, this had changed to 1:4.[39] Ideally, fully informed patients should be guided by individual unit results and quality of follow-up.

Laparoscopic gastric banding is a least-invasive operation, but does not provide as good control of diabetes as Roux-en-Y gastric bypass, biliopancreatic diversion or duodenal switch. This suggests that patients should have a choice of operation and, therefore, of referral to a unit with appropriate expertise.[34] Provided patients avoid complications, banding can lead to good weight loss, but long-term follow-up reports are lacking and its viability over time is unknown.[38] Gastric bypass has been shown to produce good weight loss durable to 15 years.[8] Biliopancreatic diversion and duodenal switch provide more weight loss at the expense of greater risk of nutritional deficiency.[33]

Key point 6

• Cultural factors, surgeon and patient preference drive choice of operation which should be based on the balance of risk and benefit.

HOSPITAL AND SURGEON VOLUME AND THE LEARNING CURVE

There are now several studies showing a clear relationship between hospital and surgeon volume and mortality after Roux-en-Y gastric bypass. Not surprisingly, inexperience has been found to be closely linked to increased operative mortality.[52] Long-term survival advantage presupposes the lowest achievable operative mortality. Just as for cancer resection and other higher risk procedures, this is a clear argument for centralisation of Roux-en-Y gastric bypass (and, by implication, biliopancreatic diversion/duodenal switch) to centres with high throughput, especially when higher risk patients are selected for surgery.[53–55] In the US, centralisation for Roux-en-Y gastric bypass does appear to be happening,[56] and surgeon volume must be 50 per year and hospital volume 125 per year to satisfy eligibility criteria to be an ASMBS 'Center of Excellence'. As the mortality for gastric banding is of the order of 0.1%, there are no data on the effect on mortality of centralisation for this operation. For all other operations, it seems important to stratify risk so that these patients have optimised outcome. Then the highest risk patients, who might benefit most, could be offered realistic survival odds from surgery compared to no surgery.[15]

Key point 7

- Better results with increased hospital and surgeon volume should drive specialisation.

COST EFFECTIVENESS

In addition to its health benefits, bariatric surgery is cost effective, with the cost of surgery being recouped within 3–4 years due to savings in treatment of on-going co-morbidities.[57,58] Costs per QALY of non-surgical treatments are more than for surgery because they fail to provide effective weight loss. Put another way, the cost per kilogram weight loss from surgery is much less than with the available medical treatments.[59]

Obesity reduces economic productivity, obese people have more days off due to illness and they have lower earnings than normal-weight people.[60] This is an important consideration as many bariatric surgery patients are young and have a large proportion of their working lives ahead of them. After surgery, more patients have paid work, they are more productive, they take fewer sick days and they rely less on state benefit.[61,62] As none of these factors have been included in traditional cost-benefit analysis, it appears that the economic advantages of bariatric surgery could be even greater than commonly supposed. In spite of this, the cost of surgery is often quoted as a major barrier to its provision.

Key point 8

- Bariatric surgery pays for itself within 3–4 years after surgery.

BARIATRIC SURGERY CONFERS LONG-TERM SURVIVAL BENEFIT

The largest prospective trial to date is the Swedish Obese Subjects study from which 15-year data are now available for over 4000 patients divided between surgery and controls.[8] The hazard ratio for death among surgery patients was 0.76 (95% confidence interval [CI], 0.59–0.99; $P = 0.04$). In a population-based study of more than 15,000 people in Utah in which driving license data were used to find matched controls, surgery (Roux-en-Y gastric bypass) provided a survival benefit of 33% at 7 years.[63] Other studies have found similarly.[64] Importantly, in the Utah study, mortality in the first year after surgery was only 0.53%, the same as the risk in the first year of not operating in the control patients, during which time 0.52% died. This implies that operative mortality must be low from Roux-en-Y gastric bypass in order to achieve long term survival benefit.

Only one paper has reported on survival benefit after gastric banding.[65] These authors found a relative risk of dying in > 800 patients of 0.36 (95% CI, 0.16–0.80; $P = 0.0004$) after 5 years compared to matched controls.

Key point 9

- Bariatric surgery patients have better long-term survival than obese controls.

CONCLUSIONS

The arguments in favour of bariatric surgery due to its cost effectiveness, reduction in co-morbidity, improved quality of life and prolonged survival appear overwhelming. Thus, on a population level, there appears to be more risk from not operating.[64]

Key point 10

- In the UK, provision of bariatric surgery by the NHS needs to increase rapidly to match other developed countries.

Those who commission health services should wholeheartedly embrace this new paradigm of care.[44] Bariatric surgery should now be considered a mainstream surgical specialty and there needs to be surgical training programmes put in place to meet the need.[34]

Key points for clinical practice

- Bariatric surgery is the only effective long-term treatment for severe obesity.

- Education and multidisciplinary assessment are essential to optimise patient preparation for surgery; commitment by the team and patient to long-term follow-up is mandatory. *(continued)*

Key points for clinical practice (continued)

- Roux-en-Y gastric bypass is the commonest operation world-wide with 60–70% excess weight loss durable to 15 years. Access for the procedure is increasingly laparoscopic.

- Gastric banding is a least-invasive operation with 50–60% excess weight loss over 5 years but long-term results are unknown and the complication rate may be cumulative.

- Roux-en-Y gastric bypass, biliopancreatic diversion and duodenal switch lead to remission of diabetes in > 80% of cases, probably by hormonal mechanism as it occurs before weight loss.

- Cultural factors, surgeon and patient preference drive choice of operation which should be based on the balance of risk and benefit.

- Better results with increased hospital and surgeon volume should drive specialisation.

- Bariatric surgery pays for itself within 3–4 years after surgery.

- Bariatric surgery patients have better long-term survival than obese controls.

- In the UK, provision of bariatric surgery by the NHS needs to increase rapidly to match other developed countries.

References

1. Friedrich MJ. Epidemic of obesity expands its spread to developing countries. *JAMA* 2002; **287**: 1382–1386.
2. DeMaria EJ. Bariatric surgery for morbid obesity. *N Engl J Med* 2007; **356**: 2176–2183.
3. Buchwald H, Avidor Y, Braunwald E *et al.* Bariatric surgery a systematic review and meta-analysis. *JAMA* 2004; **292**: 1724–1737.
4. NIH Consensus Development Panel. Gastrointestinal surgery for severe obesity. *Ann Intern Med* 1991; **115**: 956–961.
5. Fontaine KR, Redden DT, Wang C, Westfall AO, Allison DB. Years of life lost due to obesity. *JAMA* 2003; **289**: 187–193.
6. Department of Health. *Health Survey for England 2003.* <http://www.doh.gov.uk>.
7. Yanovski SZ, Yanovski AJ. Obesity. *N Engl J Med* 2002; **364**: 591–602.
8. Sjostrom L, Narbro K, Sjostrom D *et al.* Effects of bariatric surgery on mortality in Swedish obese subjects. *N Engl J Med* 2007; **357**: 741–752.
9. Buchwald H, Cowan G, Fories J. *Surgical Management of Obesity.* Philadelphia, PA: Saunders Elsevier, 2007; 1–496.
10. Ells L, Macknight N, Wilkinson JR. Obesity surgery in England; an examination of the Health Episode Statistics 1996–2005. *Obes Surg* 2007; **17**: 400–405.
11. MacLean LD, Rhode BM, Nohr CW. Late outcome of isolated gastric bypass. *Ann Surg* 2000; **231**: 524–528.
12. Ballantyne G. Measuring outcomes following bariatric surgery: weight loss parameters, improvement in co-morbid conditions, change in quality of life and patient satisfaction. *Obes Surg* 2003; **13**: 954–964.
13. Kelly J, Tarnoff M, Shikora S *et al.* Best practice recommendations for surgical care in weight loss surgery. *Obes Res* 2005; **13**: 227–233.
14. McMahon MM, Sarr MG, Clark MM *et al.* Clinical management after bariatric surgery: value of a multidisciplinary approach. *Mayo Clin Proc* 2006; **81**: S34–S45.

15. DeMaria EJ, Murr M, Byrne TK *et al.* Validation of the Obesity Surgery Mortality Risk Score in a multicenter study proves it stratifies mortality risk in patients undergoing gastric bypass for morbid obesity. *Ann Surg* 2007; **246**: 578–584.

16. Liu RC, Sabnis AA, Forsyth C *et al.* The effects of acute preoperative weight loss on laparoscopic Roux-en-Y gastric bypass. *Obes Surg* 2005; **15**: 1396–1402.

17. <www.surgicalreview.org/pcoe/tertiary/tertiary_requirements.aspx> [Accessed 19 October 2007].

18. Deitel M, Shikora SA. The development of the surgical treatment of morbid obesity. *J Am Coll Nutr* 2002; **21**: 365–371.

19. Mason E, Ito I. Gastric bypass in obesity. *Surg Clin North Am* 1967; **47**: 1345–1351.

20. Wittgrove AC, Clark W, Tremblay LJ. Laparoscopic gastric bypass, Roux en-Y: preliminary report of five cases. *Obes Surg* 1994; **4**: 353–357.

21. Nguyen NT, Goldman C, Rosenquist CJ *et al.* Laparoscopic versus open gastric bypass: a randomized study of outcomes, quality of life, and costs. *Ann Surg* 2001; **234**: 279–291.

22. Higa KD, Boone KB, Ho T. Complications of the laparoscopic Roux-en-Y gastric bypass: 1,040 patients – What have we learned? *Obes Surg* 2000; **10**: 509–513.

23. Mitchell JE, Lancaster KL, Burgard MA et el. Long-term follow-up of patients' status after gastric bypass. *Obes Surg* 2001; **11**: 464–468.

24. Christou, N, Look D, MacLean L. Weight gain after short- and long-limb gastric bypass in patients followed for longer than 10 years. *Ann Surg* 2006; **244**: 734–740.

25. Stubbs RS. Gastric bypass for severe obesity – still the gold standard: HP024. *Aust NZ J Surg* 2006; **76 (Suppl 1)**: A40.

26. White S, Brooks E, Jurikova L, Stubbs RS. Long-term outcomes after gastric bypass. *Obes Surg* 2005; **15**: 155–163.

27. Angrisani L, Lorenzo M, Borrelli V. Laparoscopic adjustable gastric banding versus Roux-en-Y gastric bypass: 5-year results of a prospective randomized trial. *SOARD* 2007; **3**: 127–133.

28. Weber M, Muller M, Bucher T *et al.* Laparoscopic gastric bypass is superior to laparoscopic gastric banding for treatment of morbid obesity. *Ann Surg* 2004; **240**: 975–983.

29. Brolin RE, Kenler HA, Gorman JH, Cody RP. Long-limb gastric bypass in the super-obese: a prospective randomised study. *Ann Surg* 1992; **215**: 387–395.

30. Bloomberg RD, Fleishman A, Nalle JE *et al.* Nutritional deficiencies following bariatric surgery: what have we learned? *Obes Surg* 2005; **15**: 145–154.

31. le Roux CW, Welbourn R, Werling M *et al.* Gut hormones as mediators of appetite and weight loss after Roux-en-Y gastric bypass. *Ann Surg* 2007; **246**: 780–785.

32. Mason EE, Doherty C, Cullen JJ, Scott D, Rodriguez EM, Maher JW. Vertical gastroplasty: evaluation of vertical banded gastroplasty. *World J Surg* 1998; **22**: 919–924.

33. Scopinaro N, Adami GF, Marinari GM *et al.* Biliopancreatic diversion. *World J Surg* 1998; **22**: 936–946.

34. Buchwald H. Overview of bariatric surgery. *J Am Coll Surg* 2002; **194**: 367–375.

35. Hess DS, Hess DW. Biliopancreatic diversion with duodenal switch. *Obes Surg* 1998; **8**: 267–282.

36. Hashemi M. Laparoscopic gastric banding for obesity. *Rec Adv Surg* 2006; **29**: 119–133.

37. Belachew M, Legrand MJ, Vincent V. History of Lap-Band: from dream to reality. *Obes Surg* 2001; **11**: 297–302.

38. O'Brien PE, McPhail T, Chaston TB, Dixon JB. Systematic review of medium-term weight loss after bariatric operations. *Obes Surg* 2006; **16**: 1032–1040.

39. Suter M, Calmes JM, Paroz A, Giusti V. A 10-year experience with laparoscopic gastric banding for morbid obesity: high long-term complication and failure rates. *Obes Surg* 2006; **16**: 829–835.

40. Weiner R, Blanco-Engert R, Weiner S, Matkowitz R, Schaefer L, Pomhoff I. Outcome after laparoscopic adjustable gastric banding – 8 years experience. *Obes Surg* 2003; **13**: 427–434.

41. Gagner M, Rogula T. Laparoscopic reoperative sleeve gastrectomy for poor weight loss after biliopancreatic diversion with duodenal switch. *Obes Surg* 2003; **13**: 649–654.

42. Johnston D, Dachtler J, Sue-Ling HM, King RF, Martin G. The Magenstrasse and Mill operation for morbid obesity. *Obes Surg* 2003; **13**: 10–16.

43. Melissas J, Mouzas J, Filis D *et al*. The intragastric balloon – smoothing the path to bariatric surgery. *Obes Surg* 2006; **16**: 897–902.

44. Dixon JB, Pories WJ, O'Brien PE, Schauer PR, Zimmet P. Surgery as an effective early intervention for diabesity. Why the reluctance? *Diabetes Care* 2005; **28**: 472–474.

45. Dymek MP, Le Grange D, Neven K, Alverdy J. Quality of life and psychological adjustment in patients after Roux-en-Y gastric bypass: a brief report. *Obes Surg* 2001; **11**: 32–39.

46. Pories WJ, Swanson MS, MacDonald KG *et al*. Who would have thought it? An operation proves to be the most effective therapy for adult-onset diabetes mellitus. *Ann Surg* 1995; **222**: 339–352.

47. Hickey MS, Pories WJ, MacDonald KG *et al*. A new paradigm for type 2 diabetes mellitus: could it be a disease of the foregut? *Ann Surg* 1998; **227**: 637–644.

48. Diabetes Surgery Summit, Rome 2007. <http://www.asbs.org/html/pdf/phil_schauer_md_letter.pdf> [Accessed 12 June 2007].

49. Schauer PR, Burguera B, Ikramuddin S *et al*. Effect of laparoscopic Roux-en-Y on type-2 diabetes mellitus. *Ann Surg* 2003; **283**: 467–485.

50. Rubino F, Forgione A, Cummings DE *et al*. The mechanism of diabetes control after gastrointestinal bypass surgery reveals a role of the proximal small intestine in the pathophysiology of type 2 diabetes. *Ann Surg* 2006; **244**: 741–749.

51. Courcoulas A, Flum D. Filling the gaps in bariatric surgical research. *JAMA* 2005; **294**: 1957–1960.

52. Flum D, Dellinger EP. Impact of gastric bypass operation on survival: a population-based analysis. *J Am Coll Surg* 2004; **11**: 543–551.

53. Nguyen NT, Paya M, Stevens CM, Mavandadi S, Zainabadi K, Wilson SE. The relationship between hospital volume and outcome in bariatric surgery at academic medical centers. *Ann Surg* 2004; **240**: 586–594.

54. Courcoulas A, Schuchert M, Gatti M *et al*. The relationship of surgeon and hospital volume to outcome after gastric bypass surgery in Pennsylvania: a 3-year summary. *Surgery* 2003; **134**: 613–623.

55. Murr MM, Taylor M, Haines K *et al*. A state-wide review of contemporary outcomes of gastric bypass in Florida: does provider volume impact outcomes? *Ann Surg* 2007; **245**: 699–706.

56. Birkmeyer N, Wei Y, Goldfaden A, Birkmeyer JD. Characteristics of hospitals performing bariatric surgery. *JAMA* 2006; **295**: 282–284.

57. Sampalis JS, Liberman M, Auger S, Christou NV. The impact of weight reduction surgery on healthcare costs in morbidly obese patients. *Obes Surg* 2004; **14**: 939–947.

58. Snow LL, Weinstein LS, Hannon JK *et al*. The effect of Roux en Y gastric bypass on prescription drug costs. *Obes Surg* 2004; **14**: 1031–1035.

59. Martin LF, Tan TL, Horn JR *et al*. Comparison of the costs associated with medical and surgical treatment of obesity. *Surgery* 1995; **118**: 599–607.

60. Suhrcke M, McKee M, Arce RS, Tsolova S, Mortensen J. Investment in health could be good for Europe's economies. *BMJ* 2006; **333**: 1017–1019.

61. Narbro K, Agren G, Jonsson E *et al*. Sick leave and disability pension before and after treatment for obesity: a report from the Swedish Obese Subjects (SOS) study. *Int J Obes* 1999; **23**: 619–624.

62. Hawkins SC, Osborne A, Finlay I *et al*. Paid work increases and state benefit claims decrease after bariatric surgery. *Obes Surg* 2007; **17**: 434–437.

63. Adams TD, Gress RE, Smith SC *et al*. Long-term mortality after gastric bypass surgery. *N Engl J Med* 2007; **357**: 753–761.

64. <www.asbs.org/Newsite07/resources/asmbs_items.htm> [Accessed 19 October 2007].

65. Busetto, L, Mirabelli D, Petroni ML *et al*. Comparative long-term mortality after laparoscopic adjustable gastric banding versus nonsurgical controls. *SOARD* 2007; **3**: 496–502.

Sangeeta A. Paisey Andrew R. Bateman

6

Neoadjuvant chemoradiotherapy for pancreatic cancer

Adenocarcinoma of the pancreas has an appalling prognosis. The majority of patients present with metastatic or locally advanced inoperable disease. Surgery remains the mainstay of radical treatment in the 10–20% of presenting patients suitable for resection. Despite resection, median survival times are poor and long-term survivors few.[1] Neoadjuvant chemoradiotherapy is an approach which may improve outcomes in patients with resectable or potentially resectable pancreatic cancer. However, there are no prospective, randomised, Phase III trials for neoadjuvant treatment of pancreatic cancer and the data in support of its use are from non-randomised series. Here we discuss the use of neoadjuvant chemoradiotherapy in resectable tumours and extend the discussion to include the role of chemoradiotherapy in inoperable, locally advanced, non-metastatic, pancreatic cancer.

The annual incidence of pancreatic cancer is approximately 100 per million population; it is the sixth most common cause of cancer death in the UK and US.[2] Potentially curative resection is only possible in 10–20% of patients. However, the 5-year overall survival even with radical resection is still only 20% in the best centres,[3] with the median survival after R0 resection in the region of 14–25 months.[4] On a more positive note, mortality from surgery has dropped significantly over the last few decades from 25% to less than 5%. This is due to a combination of factors including better patient selection, high-dependency care postoperatively, and centralisation of patients to regional surgical centres.[5–7]

Sangeeta A. Paisey MBBS MRCP(UK)
Specialist Registrar Clinical Oncology, Cancer Care Directorate, Mail Point 301, Level B, Southampton General Hospital, Southampton SO16 6YD, UK
E-mail: sangeeta@doctors.org.uk

Andrew R. Bateman MRCP FRCR PhD (for correspondence)
Senior Lecturer/Honorary Consultant Clinical Oncologist, University of Sourgampton, Somers Cancers Sciences Building MP824, Southampton General Hospital, Southampton SO16 6YD, UK
E-mail: Andrew.Bateman@suht.swest.nhs.uk

The patterns of failure after surgical resection are primarily intra-abdominal, with pancreatic bed, hepatic and peritoneal recurrence accounting for over 90% of the total. This pattern of relapse, coupled with the frequency of lymphatic spread (75% of cases), is used to support the rationale for multimodality treatment approaches, whether adjuvant or neoadjuvant, to complement surgery and improve outcomes.

ADJUVANT THERAPY

The current UK standard of care has been to offer suitable patients (R0–1 resection, reasonable performance status) adjuvant chemotherapy. This is based on the results of the European Study Group for Pancreatic Cancer (ESPAC) I trial.[8] The ESPAC 1 trial[9] was a randomised study of 541 patients comparing adjuvant treatment with chemotherapy and/or chemoradiotherapy versus observation alone. There was evidence of a survival benefit for 5-fluoro-uracil (5-FU)-based adjuvant chemotherapy with a median survival of 19·7 months with chemotherapy and 14·0 months without. A median survival of 15·5 months with chemoradiotherapy versus 16·1 months without suggested no benefit for adjuvant chemoradiotherapy. It should be noted that this trial has received considerable criticism, particularly from the US, in part due to the randomisation process involved,[10] but also due to the use of an antiquated radiotherapy schedule and technique, and lack of radiotherapy quality assurance. That being said, the study conclusion that adjuvant 5-FU chemotherapy improves outcomes has been widely adopted in Europe.

As gemcitabine is the most effective single agent in metastatic disease,[11] it is clearly important to define its effect in the adjuvant setting. The first randomised Phase III trial in patients with resected pancreatic cancer has recently been published (CONKO – 001).[12] This study again randomised to adjuvant therapy versus observation alone. The study demonstrated a statistically significant difference in disease-free survival of 14.2 months in the gemcitabine arm to 7.5 months in the observation arm. However, no overall survival advantage was demonstrated due to patients in the observation arm receiving gemcitabine on progression suggesting that the timing of chemotherapy may not be crucial.

Defining which chemotherapy agent (5-FU or gemcitabine) is optimum as adjuvant therapy should be answered by the current European Phase III study, ESPAC 3, which has recently completed accrual. Patients with curative resection of pancreatic cancer were randomised to 5-FU + folinic acid versus gemcitabine (a third observation-only arm was dropped following data review).[13]

In the US, adjuvant chemoradiation is still considered standard treatment following earlier studies, particularly the 'landmark' trial conducted by the Gastrointestinal Tumor Study Group (GITSG).[14] A recent Radiation Therapy Oncology Group (RTOG) 9704 trial was designed to test gemcitabine before and after standard chemoradiotherapy (50.4 Gy plus 5-FU) versus 5-FU before and after standard chemoradiotherapy. Of the 538 patients recruited, 442 were eligible for analysis. A modest, but significant, improved survival was observed in patients with tumours of the pancreatic head who received gemcitabine (n = 380), with a median survival of 18.8 months for the gemcitabine arm versus 16.7 months for the 5-FU arm, and 3-year survival of 31% versus 21%, respectively.[15] Overall, there was no significant difference in survival when analysis included the patients with tumours of the body and tail of the pancreas.

Thus far, studies including ESPAC and GITSG have shown an increased median survival in patients who received adjuvant treatment when compared with those treated with surgery alone. Which modalities, specific agents and combinations continue to be an area of research and debate.

Key point 1

- The current standard of care in the UK is surgery followed by adjuvant chemotherapy (adjuvant chemoradiotherapy in the US).

NEOADJUVANT THERAPY

Neoadjuvant treatment has been demonstrated to be effective and has become routine practice in a number of gastrointestinal tumour sites: including oesophagus, gastric[5] and rectal cancer,[5,16,17] and will soon be examined in a Phase III study in colon cancer in the UK (FOxTROT). The theoretical advantages for introducing either chemotherapy or chemoradiotherapy early in the therapeutic pathway, before surgery, are common to all disease sites. The advantages include:

1. Early introduction of systemic and regional treatment down-stages the pancreatic tumour resulting in improved R0 resection rate[18,19] and decreasing the rate of positive metastatic lymph nodes (from 60–80%[6,20–22] in untreated resections to 30–48% after neoadjuvant chemoradiotherapy.[23,24]

2. Better tolerability for chemotherapy/chemoradiotherapy when given pre-operatively.[25] Only 40–60% of patients after pancreatic resection receive adjuvant treatment due to slow or incomplete recovery from surgery, or through patients declining further treatment after a major operative intervention.

3. With respect to chemoradiotherapy, there are radiobiological advantages of pre-operative chemoradiotherapy over postoperative treatment. These include: (i) reduced chance of tumour hypoxia with neoadjuvant treatment (hypoxia is a well-known mechanism of chemoradiotherapy resistance[26]); (ii) reduction in mucosal and anastomotic toxicity;[27,28] and (iii) avoidance of the potential for tumour repopulation as a result of delay in radiation delivery after surgery.

4. A period of observation for patients receiving neoadjuvant treatment prior to surgery allows those with particularly aggressive tumours and occult metastatic disease to manifest themselves; this avoids futile non-therapeutic resections.

These theoretical advantages for neoadjuvant treatment have been apparent for some considerable time. Due to the nature of pancreatic cancer, neoadjuvant chemoradiotherapy has been favoured rather than chemotherapy alone. Consequently, larger centres and co-operative groups started developing Phase I/II protocols in the late 1980s and early 1990s. A representative chemoradiotherapy strategy is illustrated in Figure 1. The reports from these non-randomised, mainly single, institutional series, are of interest.

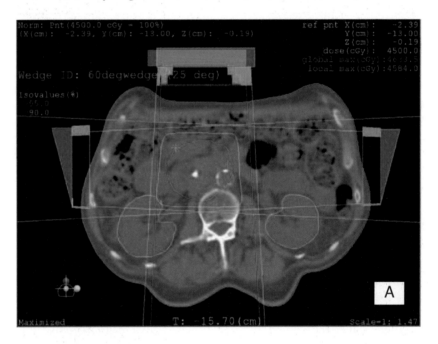

Fig. 1 Modern chemoradiotherapy protocols involve 3-D conformal radiotherapy planning and delivery. Patients are scanned in the appropriate treatment position. Axial images are obtained at 3–5 mm intervals and the tumour margin outlined. The treatment volume (planning target volume) is then defined and suitable field arrangements applied. Shielding (now commonly performed by multileaf collimators) permits maximum conforming to the treatment volume, minimising radiation dose to normal structures. Treatment may be given in two phases: phase 1, 45 Gy in 25 fractions over 5 weeks; phase 2, 5.4–10.8 Gy in 5–10 fractions over 1–2 weeks to a reduced volume. Chemotherapy is given concurrently with radiotherapy: 5-FU, gemcitabine, and cisplatin have all been incorporated in a variety of protocols. Surgery is planned to occur 6 weeks after completion of chemoradiotherapy to allow acute reactions to settle and restaging to be performed. (A) Axial view demonstrating the planning target volume (red), representative field arrangements with shielding, and critical normal structures (kidneys) outlined. (B) Sagittal view demonstrating the tumour volume (green), planning target volume (red), anterior field and representative radiotherapy dose contours (blue 95%, yellow 90%). (C) Multiplane 3-D reconstructed view.

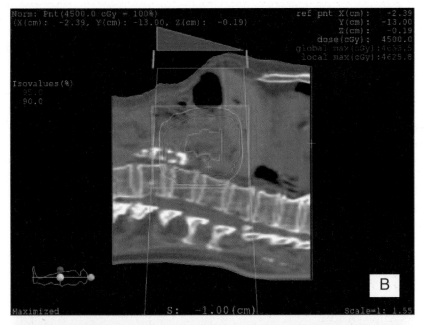

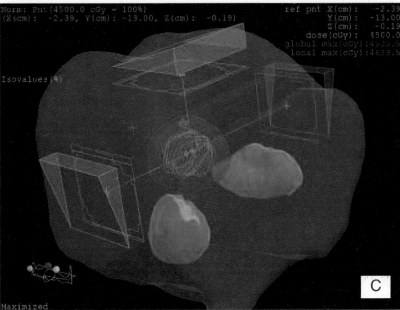

The MD Anderson group was one of the first to publish a large series.[23] They evaluated different neoadjuvant treatment schedules in 132 patients treated consecutively with pre-operative chemoradiotherapy followed by surgery, in a series beginning in 1990. Patients received concomitant chemoradiotherapy using a fairly standard radiotherapy schedule of 50.4 Gy in 28 fractions (5.5 weeks) or a short-course schedule of 30.0 Gy in 10 fractions (2 weeks); both schedules were combined with infusional chemotherapy followed by surgical resection (with [56%] or without [44%] intra-operative radiation therapy [IORT]). No adjuvant treatment was given. Eighty-eight patients received the short-course schedule. The overall median survival was 21 months and 5-year survival was 23%. Of the patients included in this series, 27% had undergone attempted resection in another centre and 43% required vascular resection and reconstruction. Despite this extensive surgery, peri-operative deaths were only 2%. Female sex and lymph node negativity were positively correlated with survival; choice of radiotherapy schedule or IORT was not a prognostic factor. Local recurrence as first site of relapse was 8%.[23]

Pendurthi[21] reported a retrospective analysis of 70 patients with pancreatic adenocarcinoma treated with either pre-operative or postoperative chemoradiation between 1986 and 1996. In the adjuvant therapy group, 22% did not receive treatment for various reasons. Review of histology showed significantly fewer involved nodes in the neoadjuvant treatment group (28% versus 87%), and increased number of R0 resections (28 versus 56%). Toxicities and survival were comparable in both groups.[21]

Coia[22] reported a small, prospective study. Pathological nodal response and surgical clearance were assessed in 31 patients after pre-operative chemoradiotherapy for adenocarcinoma of the pancreas or duodenum. Of these, 27 patients had pancreatic cancer, and four patients had carcinoma of the duodenum. A total dose of 50.4 Gy in 1.8 Gy per fraction was delivered concurrently with two cycles of chemotherapy with a 4-day infusion of 5-FU on days 2 and 29, and mitomycin-C on day 2 only, followed 4–6 weeks later by surgical resection. Of 31 patients, 29 completed the entire pre-operative regimen and 55% underwent curative resection. Only 2 of 17 had pathologic nodal involvement, none with involved margins. The conclusion was that concomitant chemoradiotherapy for cancer of the pancreas was a well-tolerated therapy that down-staged nodal metastases and improved R0 resection rates.[22] The 3-year survival in this study was high and is currently being evaluated in a larger Phase II trial.

An outcomes trial between 1989 and 1997, reported by Snady,[29] aimed to determine the benefit of chemoradiotherapy prior to surgery in 159 consecutive patients with localised pancreatic tumours: 68 patients were deemed inoperable at presentation and received split course radiotherapy with 5-FU, streptozotocin and cisplatin followed by surgery in down-staged patients (20 of 68). Ninety-one operable patients underwent initial surgical resection followed by adjuvant chemotherapy with or without radiotherapy. The 30-day postoperative mortality rate was nil for the chemoradiotherapy group and 5% for the initially operable group. The overall survival was 23.6 months in the chemoradiotherapy group and 14 months in the patients receiving adjuvant therapy. The conclusion from this study suggested that chemoradiotherapy was able to reverse the expected trend that patients with earlier stage disease should have a better prognosis.

Sasson[30] reported a retrospective analysis of 116 patients with pancreatic cancer who underwent resection at Fox Chase Cancer Center between 1987 and 2000. In total, 53% of these patients received pre-operative chemotherapy, with 5-FU/MMC or gemcitabine, concurrently with external beam radio-therapy (50.4 Gy). Pathology was compared between patients receiving neoadjuvant chemoradiotherapy and those proceeding straight to surgery. The amount of fibrosis present in the tumour (relative to the amount of neoplastic cells) was significantly higher after administration of pre-operative treatment. Higher fibrosis levels were associated with negative lymph nodes and negative margins. The median survival was similarly better in the neoadjuvant group – 23 months versus 16 months without.[30]

White *et al.*[24] described the Duke experience where 193 patients with local pancreatic cancer were treated with neoadjuvant chemoradiotherapy between 1994 and 2004. This series included potentially resectable (102 patients) and 91 patients deemed initially unresectable. Exact chemoradiotherapy treatments varied but 95% received 5-FU-based schedules with 50.4 Gy in 28 fractions radiotherapy. Overall, 54 of 102 (53%) and 16 of 91 (18%) patients underwent resection with a 4.5% 30-day postoperative mortality. Median survival for all resected patients was 22 months and the 5-year overall survival was 27%. The figures for the potentially resectable group only were median survival of 39 months and 5-year overall survival of 40%.

Key points 3–5

- The benefit of neoadjuvant chemoradiotherapy has not yet been demonstrated in a randomised trial but is currently being evaluated. This emphasises the need for appropriate trial development and recruitment of patients into clinical trials.

- Neoadjuvant chemoradiotherapy increases the number of patients receiving all-treatment modalities.

- Neoadjuvant chemoradiotherapy improves R0 resection rates and reduces node positivity.

In a detailed pathological analysis, lymph node status after chemo-radiotherapy was confirmed to be an important prognostic feature; lymph node negative (70%) had a 12-month improved median overall survival compared to lymph node positive patients. Tumour differentiation, extent of necrosis and residual tumour load were all inversely associated with survival. Interestingly, radiographic response to chemoradiotherapy was not helpful, presumably due to the extensive fibrosis seen after chemoradiotherapy in many cases. Epithelial growth factor receptor (EGFR) over-expression was only identified in 5% of specimens after chemoradiotherapy, whereas p53 over-expression was identified in 44% but this was not an independent prognostic factor.

An interesting, but small, study was recently reported by a Finnish group.[31] Here, 47 consecutive patients with operable pancreatic carcinoma were entered into a non-randomised study of pre-operative chemoradiotherapy or proceeded straight to surgery. Selection was based on whether the patients were local to the hospital (chemoradiotherapy group) or lived some distance away (surgery only group). On staging criteria, the two cohorts were evenly matched. Chemoradiotherapy consisted of gemcitabine given synchronously with 50.4 Gy in 28 fractions. Adjuvant chemotherapy was not given in the study.

Of the 22 who received chemoradiotherapy, eight did not undergo surgery due to development of metastatic disease or deterioration in performance status. Overall, there was no difference in survival between the two groups. Operative mortality was 2% and morbidity was not significantly different.

Key point 6

- Use of neoadjuvant therapy up front identifies patients with occult metastases (thus avoiding unnecessary surgery) and provides appropriate palliative treatment.

In summary, the conclusions that can be drawn from the available literature regarding neoadjuvant chemoradiotherapy in operable pancreatic cancer are:

1. A number of chemoradiation schedules have been described and tested which are reasonably well tolerated and do not lead to significant increased postoperative morbidity or mortality. The majority of patients complete all modalities of treatment.

2. Accurate staging/assessment of operability and histological confirmation are imperative for appropriate decision making in treatment. After chemoradiotherapy, assessment can be difficult due to treatment-induced fibrosis.

3. A significant proportion of patients receiving neoadjuvant chemoradiotherapy will exhibit metastatic disease at completion, prior to surgery. This group will have received appropriate local palliation (chemoradiotherapy) and will avoid an unhelpful major surgical intervention.

4. The survival data from neoadjuvant studies are sufficiently encouraging, relative to standard of care, to advocate recruitment to carefully designed randomised trials of chemoradiotherapy prior to surgery.

With regard to the final comment, a German co-operative group has developed such a study.[32] The study is a multicentre. randomised, Phase III trial. All participating centres offer modern 3-D conformal radiotherapy and conduct more than 15 pancreaticoduodenectomies per year. Patients with operable ductal adenocarcinoma of the pancreatic head will be randomised to primary resection (partial duodenopancreatectomy with defined lymphatic dissection) or neoadjuvant chemoradiotherapy followed by surgery. All patients will receive adjuvant gemcitabine. The neoadjuvant chemoradiotherapy consists of 55.8 Gy in 31 fractions concomitantly with gemcitabine and cisplatin. The primary outcome measure will be overall survival with secondary outcome measures including quality of life, *etc.*

ROLE OF CHEMORADIOTHERAPY IN BORDERLINE/MARGINALLY RESECTABLE PANCREATIC CANCER

As indicated in some of the previously described series, within the group of non-metastatic pancreatic cancers, some tumours will be borderline operable or unresectable. In retrospective series this is a difficult area to clarify due to the variation in staging techniques and discrepancy between groups as to what constitutes operable/inoperable disease. However, it is important to clarify what neoadjuvant chemoradiotherapy may offer to this group of patients. A representative study, which addresses this issue, is from an Italian group.[33] They reported their experience of patients treated between 1999 and 2003 using modern imaging equipment, enabling clear definition of the superior mesenteric vessels, portal vein and celiac axis. Borderline cases were defined as having vein stenosis or arterial abutment ($n = 18$), unresectable as having vein thrombosis or arterial encasement ($n = 10$). All patients received chemoradiotherapy and were restaged. Responding patients, or those with stable disease and Ca19.9 in the normal range, were surgically explored. Only one unresectable tumour was successfully resected compared to 7 out of 18 (39%) that were borderline resectable. Survival for resected patients was equivalent to patients with operable tumours at presentation, with only those patients with an R0 resection having disease survival longer than 24 months.

Key point 7

- Neoadjuvant chemoradiotherapy combined with surgery may improve local control. However, this approach will most likely need to be combined with improved systemic treatment to demonstrate marked improvement in survival rates.

LOCALLY ADVANCED INOPERABLE PANCREATIC CANCER

Patients with locally advanced inoperable pancreatic cancers have historically been included into studies containing patients with metastatic disease. Consequently, it is not clear whether this group should receive chemotherapy alone or may benefit from chemoradiotherapy. The FFCD-SRFO study[34] recently published the results of a randomised Phase III trial focusing on locally advanced tumours. The study compared chemoradiotherapy with 60 Gy (with concomitant 5-FU and cisplatin treatment) followed by sequential gemcitabine versus gemcitabine induction and maintenance. The survival was significantly lower in patients with initial chemoradiotherapy – 8.4 months versus 14.3 months in the chemotherapy arm. These data led to the study being terminated prematurely because of the lower survival in the initial chemoradiotherapy arm. The conclusions drawn by the authors were that gemcitabine alone was sufficient in improving overall survival in locally advanced, non-metastatic, pancreatic cancer. However, there is no doubt that the dose of radiotherapy prescribed in the study was too high; this is borne out by the high levels of gastrointestinal and haematological toxicities seen in the chemoradiotherapy cohort.

Huguet et al.[35] conducted a retrospective review of 181 locally advanced patients enrolled in recent Groupe Cooperateur Multidisciplinaire en Oncologie (GERCOR) prospective Phase II and III chemotherapy studies. The prospective studies were designed to assess chemotherapy regimens in both metastatic and locally advanced pancreatic cancer. After 3 months, responding or stable patients with locally advanced tumours were recommended to receive chemoradiotherapy.

The median overall survival for the 181 patients was 11.4 months. About 29% of these patients developed metastatic disease after 3 months of induction chemotherapy. Of the 128 remaining patients, 72 (56%) received chemoradio-therapy and 56 (44%) maintenance chemotherapy at the discretion of their treatment teams. The overall survival was significantly better in the chemoradiotherapy group – 15 months versus 11.7 months.

A randomised Phase III trial conducted by the GERCOR and AIO groups is currently evaluating this strategy of induction chemotherapy followed by chemoradiotherapy in non-progressors, and a UK study (SCALP) is in the advanced stage of set-up.

CONCLUSIONS

Pancreatic cancer remains one of the sternest challenges to cancer management. Improvements in outcomes have been made by centralisation of services to specialist centres. This has led to improved patient assessment, selection and improved surgical outcomes. However, the median overall survival and the number of long-term survivors following surgical resection alone remains poor. The addition of adjuvant treatment has had some incremental benefit. The theoretical advantages and experience of neoadjuvant chemoradiotherapy to date has been highlighted. Initial clarification of the role, if any, for neoadjuvant chemoradiotherapy awaits the outcome from randomised Phase III studies. Optimisation of radiotherapy and chemotherapy schedules, and combinations will require careful trial design and study for what will be a highly complex patient pathway.

Key points for clinical practice

- The current standard of care in the UK is surgery followed by adjuvant chemotherapy (adjuvant chemoradiotherapy in the US).

- Neoadjuvant chemoradiotherapy is an attractive approach to improve outcomes in selected patients with operable or borderline operable pancreatic cancer.

- The benefit of neoadjuvant chemoradiotherapy has not yet been demonstrated in a randomised trial but is currently being evaluated. This emphasises the need for appropriate trial development and recruitment of patients into clinical trials.

- Neoadjuvant chemoradiotherapy increases the number of patients receiving all-treatment modalities.

- Neoadjuvant chemoradiotherapy improves R0 resection rates and reduces node positivity.

- Use of neoadjuvant therapy up front identifies patients with occult metastases (thus avoiding unnecessary surgery) and provides appropriate palliative treatment.

- Neoadjuvant chemoradiotherapy combined with surgery may improve local control. However, this approach will most likely need to be combined with improved systemic treatment to demonstrate marked improvement in survival rates.

References

1. Carpelan-Holmstrom M, Nordling S, Pukkala E *et al*. Does anyone survive pancreatic ductal adenocarcinoma? A nationwide study re-evaluating the data of the Finnish Cancer Registry. *Gut* 2005; **54**: 385–387.
2. Gold EB. Epidemiology of and risk factors for pancreatic cancer. *Surg Clin North Am* 1995; **75**: 819–843.
3. Richter A, Niedergethmann M, Sturm JW, Lorenz D, Post S, Trede M. Long-term results of partial pancreaticoduodenectomy for ductal adenocarcinoma of the pancreatic head: 25-year experience. *World J Surg* 2003; **27**: 324–329.
4. Hohenberger W, Kastl S. [Neoadjuvant and adjuvant therapy of ductal pancreatic carcinoma]. *Zentralbl Chir* 2000; **125**: 348–355.
5. Medical Research Council Oesophageal Cancer Working Group. Surgical resection with or without preoperative chemotherapy in oesophageal cancer: a randomised controlled trial. *Lancet* 2002; **359**: 1727–1733.
6. Sohn TA, Yeo CJ, Cameron JL *et al*. Resected adenocarcinoma of the pancreas-616 patients: results, outcomes, and prognostic indicators. *J Gastrointest Surg* 2000; **4**: 567–579.
7. Yeo CJ, Cameron JL, Sohn TA *et al*. Six hundred fifty consecutive pancreaticoduodenectomies in the 1990s: pathology, complications, and outcomes. *Ann Surg* 1997; **226**: 248–257.
8. Neoptolemos JP, Stocken DD, Friess H *et al*. A randomized trial of chemoradiotherapy and chemotherapy after resection of pancreatic cancer. *N Engl J Med* 2004; **350**: 1200–1210.
9. Neoptolemos JP, Dunn JA, Stocken DD *et al*. Adjuvant chemoradiotherapy and chemotherapy in resectable pancreatic cancer: a randomised controlled trial. *Lancet* 2001; **358**: 1576–1585.
10. Abrams RA, Lillemoe KD, Piantadosi S. Continuing controversy over adjuvant therapy of pancreatic cancer. *Lancet* 2001; **358**: 1565–1566.
11. Burris III HA. Recent updates on the role of chemotherapy in pancreatic cancer. *Semin Oncol* 2005; **32 (Suppl 6)**: S1–S3.
12. Oettle H, Post S, Neuhaus P *et al*. Adjuvant chemotherapy with gemcitabine vs observation in patients undergoing curative-intent resection of pancreatic cancer: a randomized controlled trial. *JAMA* 2007; **297**: 267–277.
13. Owen E. *ESPAC-3(v2) Adjuvant Chemotherapies in Resectable Pancreatic Cancer*. The University of Liverpool. Division of Surgery and Oncology, 2007.
14. Kalser MH, Ellenberg SS. Pancreatic cancer. Adjuvant combined radiation and chemotherapy following curative resection. *Arch Surg* 1985; **120**: 899–903.
15. ASCO Annual Meeting Proceedings. *J Clin Oncol* 2006; **24 (Suppl 18)**.
16. Cunningham D, Allum WH, Stenning SP *et al*. Perioperative chemotherapy versus surgery alone for resectable gastroesophageal cancer. *N Engl J Med* 2006; **355**: 11–20.
17. Sauer R, Becker H, Hohenberger W *et al*. Preoperative versus postoperative chemoradiotherapy for rectal cancer. *N Engl J Med* 2004; **351**: 1731–1740.
18. Pingpank JF, Hoffman JP, Ross EA *et al*. Effect of preoperative chemoradiotherapy on surgical margin status of resected adenocarcinoma of the head of the pancreas. *J Gastrointest Surg* 2001; **5**: 121–130.
19. Snady H, Bruckner H, Siegel J, Cooperman A, Neff R, Kiefer L. Endoscopic ultrasonographic criteria of vascular invasion by potentially resectable pancreatic tumors. *Gastrointest Endosc* 1994; **40**: 326–333.
20. Niedergethmann A. Prognostic implications of routine, immunohistochemical, and molecular staging in resectable pancreatic adenocarcinoma. *Am J Surg Pathol* 2002; **26**: 1578–1587.
21. Pendurthi TK. Preoperative versus postoperative chemoradiation for patients with resected pancreatic adenocarcinoma. *Am Surg* 1998; **64**: 686–692.
22. Coia L. Preoperative chemoradiation for adenocarcinoma of the pancreas and duodenum. *Int J Radiat Oncol Biol Phys* 1994; **30**: 161–167.
23. Breslin TM. Neoadjuvant chemoradiotherapy for adenocarcinoma of the pancreas: treatment variables and survival duration. *Ann Surg Oncol* 2001; **8**: 123–132.

24. White RR, Xie HB, Gottfried MR *et al*. Significance of histological response to preoperative chemoradiotherapy for pancreatic cancer. *Ann Surg Oncol* 2005; **12**: 214–221.
25. Wayne JD, Wolff RA, Pisters PW, Evans DB. Multimodality management of localized pancreatic cancer. *Cancer J* 2001; **7 (Suppl 1)**: S35–S46.
26. Evans DB, Rich TA, Byrd DR *et al*. Preoperative chemoradiation and pancreaticoduodenectomy for adenocarcinoma of the pancreas. *Arch Surg* 1992; **127**: 1335–1339.
27. Pilepich MV, Miller HH. Preoperative irradiation in carcinoma of the pancreas. *Cancer* 1980; **46**: 1945–1949.
28. Wanebo HJ, Glicksman AS, Vezeridis MP *et al*. Preoperative chemotherapy, radiotherapy, and surgical resection of locally advanced pancreatic cancer. *Arch Surg* 2000; **135**: 81–87.
29. Snady H. Survival advantage of combined chemoradiotherapy compared with resection as the initial treatment of patients with regional pancreatic carcinoma. An outcomes trial. *Cancer* 2000; **89**: 314–327.
30. Sasson AR. Neoadjuvant chemoradiotherapy for adenocarcinoma of the pancreas: analysis of histopathology and outcome. *Int J Gastrointest Cancer* 2003; **34**: 121–128.
31. Vento P, Mustonen H, Joensuu T, Karkkainen P, Kivilaakso E, Kiviluoto T. Impact of preoperative chemoradiotherapy on survival in patients with resectable pancreatic cancer. *World J Gastroenterol* 2007; **13**: 2945–2951.
32. Brunner TB, Hohenberger W, Sauer R, Golcher H, Meyer T, Grabenbauer GG. Primary resection versus neoadjuvant chemoradiation followed by resection for locally resectable or potentially resectable pancreatic carcinoma without distant metastasis. A multi-centre prospectively randomised Phase II-study of the Interdisciplinary Working Group Gastrointestinal Tumours (AIO, ARO, and CAO). *BMC Cancer* 2007; **6**: 41.
33. Massucco P, Capussotti L, Magnino A *et al*. Pancreatic resections after chemoradiotherapy for locally advanced ductal adenocarcinoma: analysis of perioperative outcome and survival. *Ann Surg Oncol* 2006; **13**: 1201–1208.
34. Chauffert B. Phase III trial comparing initial chemoradiotherapy (intermittent cisplatin and infusional 5-FU) followed by gemcitabine versus gemcitabine alone in patients with locally advanced non metastatic pancreatic cancer: a FFCD–SFRO study. *J Clin Oncol* 2006; **24 (Suppl 18)**, 4008.
35. Huguet F. Impact of chemoradiotherapy after disease control with chemotherapy in locally advanced pancreatic adenocarcinoma in GERCOR Phase II and III studies. *J Clin Oncol* 2007; **25**: 326–331.

Mohammad Abu Hilal Lashan Peiris
Roberto Salvia

7

Intraductal papillary mucinous neoplasms of the pancreas

Intraductal papillary mucinous neoplasms (IPMNs) were first described by Ohashi in 1982 as 'mucin secreting cancer of the pancreas'. More recently, IPMNs have become more commonly diagnosed, even in asymptomatic patients. In certain centres, IPMNs have become the second most common indication for pancreatic resection, after ductal adenocarcinoma.[1,2] This has led to a clear improvement in the clinical, radiological and pathological understanding of the characteristics of IPMNs.[3]

The World Health Organization (WHO) has defined IPMNs as 'intraductal papillary mucinous neoplasm with tall, columnar, mucin-containing epithelium, with or without papillary projections, involving the main pancreatic duct and/or the branch ducts'.

EPIDEMIOLOGY

The recent increase in the diagnosis of IPMNs is due to two main reasons: first, a significant increase in incidentally discovered 'cystic lesions' of the pancreas; second, the inclusion of this tumour under the heading of IPMN and the consensus decision of clinicians to use this new terminology. In fact, in retrospect, it is clear that IPMN was present even before 1982 but was misclassified as mucinous cystic neoplasms or mucinous ductal cancers.

Mohammad Abu Hilal MD (for correspondence)
Consultant Hepatobiliary Pancreatic and Laparoscopic Surgeon, Honorary Senior Lecturer, School of Medicine, Southampton University Hospital, Southampton, UK
E-mail: abu_hlal@yahoo.com

Lashan Peiris MRCS
Surgical Registrar, Southampton University Hospital, Southampton, UK

Roberto Salvia MD PhD
Consultant Pancreatic Surgeon, Verona University Hospital, Verona, Italy

The incidence of IPMN peaks in the seventh and eighth decades of life; however, it is not uncommon in the fifth and sixth decades. Large series have shown that the male:female ratio is about 1:1.

Key point 1

- The incidence of IPMNs has increased significantly in the last decade due to improvement in the radiological diagnosis and better understanding and correct classification of this disease.

PATHOLOGY AND MOLECULAR BIOLOGY

In 2000, the WHO subclassified IPMNs into two different entities – main-duct IPMNs and branch-duct IPMNs. Main-duct IPMNs are characterised by involvement of the main pancreatic duct with or without associated involvement of the branch ducts (combined IPMNs).[2] Main-duct IPMN usually presents as a dilated (≥ 1 cm) main pancreatic duct full of mucus that may extrude through a bulging ampulla, even though it may look to represent a 'cyst' along the main pancreatic duct.[4]

Branch-duct IPMN involves the side branches of the pancreatic ductal system, appearing as a cystic lesion communicating with a non-dilated main pancreatic duct. The communication may be macroscopically demonstrable, which is usually dependent on the volume of mucus produced.

Three-quarters of main-duct IPMNs are located in the proximal portion of the gland; however, they have a tendency to spread to the rest of the main pancreatic duct. Branch-duct IPMNs more commonly involve the uncinate process, but they can be seen in the head, neck and distal pancreas. Multifocal involvement of the gland with two or more branch-duct IPMNs is a common finding.[1]

IPMNs may be histologically classified into benign (adenoma and borderline) and malignant (*in situ* carcinoma and invasive carcinoma); metastasis occurs in IPMNs with invasive carcinoma.

A recent review by Tanaka *et al.*[2] found that main-duct and branch-duct IPMNs were associated with malignancy in 70% and 25% of the cases, respectively, while the rate of invasive carcinoma was 43% for main-duct IPMN and 15% for branch-duct type. The biological behaviour of these two neoplasms seems to be significantly different, which affects clinical decision-making with regard to the appropriate management of these two entities.

Key point 2

- Main-duct IPMNs are more frequently associated with malignancy and invasive carcinoma. Differentiation between main- and branch-duct IPMNs is essential for correct clinical decision-making.

Different degrees of dysplasia can sometimes be recognised within the same surgical specimen; moreover, in our experience, the average age of patients with malignant main-duct IPMN is 6.4 years older than that of patients with adenoma or borderline tumour.[5] These observations support the theory of a 'clonal progression' to malignancy in this variant.[6]

Considering the molecular biology of these neoplasms, mutations in the K-ras, p16 and p53 genes are present but are less common in IPMNs than in ductal carcinoma, and DPC4 loss is usually not detected. Wada et al.[6] showed in 23 cases of resected IPMNs that two-thirds had K-ras mutation; moreover, they showed that the loss of heterozygosity in 9p21 (p16) increased from 12.5% in adenomas to 75% for carcinomas while loss of heterozygosity in 17p13 (p53) was present only in invasive carcinomas. These results suggest that loss of heterozygosity in 9p21 (p16) was an 'early' event while loss of heterozygosity in 17p13 (p53) is a later event, further supporting the theory of 'clonal progression'.

MUC proteins are a heterogeneous family of glycoproteins, some of which are located within the cell membrane and others excreted as secretory products. MUC expression profiles of IPMNs have not been clearly characterised yet. MUC1 expression, however, has been found to be associated with pancreaticobiliary type papillae and tubular carcinomas whereas MUC2 expression has been associated with intestinal type and colloid carcinoma, which has a more indolent course.

CLINICAL PRESENTATION

Patients with main-duct IPMNs are often symptomatic, being afflicted by abdominal pain, pancreatitis, steatorrhea and, less commonly, jaundice, diabetes and weight loss.[5,7–9] Even though patients affected by branch-duct IPMN can present with abdominal pain, pancreatitis or other symptoms, a large proportion of them are completely asymptomatic and neoplasms are detected incidentally during radiological investigation of other systems.[10–12] IPMN can present with a similar clinical and radiological picture as chronic pancreatitis.[13] A retrospective analysis has shown that epidemiological characteristics such as age, sex, alcohol intake and cigarette smoking differ between IPMN and chronic pancreatitis. This same study suggests that, in most cases, clinically and pathologically IPMN is the cause of chronic pancreatitis, and not vice versa.[14]

Key points 3 & 4

- Main-duct IPMNs are more likely to present with symptoms such as abdominal pain, pancreatitis, steatorrhea and, less commonly, jaundice, diabetes and weight loss.

- Branch-duct IPMNs can present with abdominal pain or pancreatitis. A large proportion of them, however, are asymptomatic and neoplasms are detected incidentally during radiological investigation of other systems.

Unlike pancreatic adenocarcinoma, jaundice is an uncommon presentation and occurs in about 15–20% of patients. Jaundice and steatorrhea at presentation should alert the physician to a much higher prevalence of malignant IPMN (8- and 5- fold, respectively). Recent onset or worsening diabetes is more common in IPMNs with invasive carcinoma (3-fold). Interestingly, anecdotal evidence suggests that patients with benign IPMNs have a higher frequency of abdominal pain and a longer duration of symptoms.

DIAGNOSTIC WORK-UP

Traditionally, the diagnosis of IPMN was made after an endoscopic retrograde cholangiopancreatography (ERCP; Fig. 1), which showed the 'triad' of Ohashi: a bulging ampulla of Vater, mucin secretion, and dilated main pancreatic duct.

Currently, the great majority of IPMNs are characterised with cross-sectional imaging with either computed tomography (CT; Fig 2) or magnetic

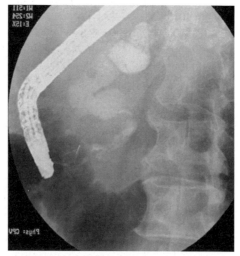

Fig. 1 Endoscopic retrograde cholangiopancreatography showing cystic dilatation of the main pancreatic duct.

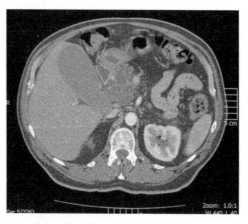

Fig. 2 Computed Tomography showing a multicystic septated mass replacing the head of the pancreas representing a large combined type IPMN

A

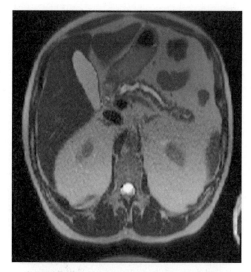

B

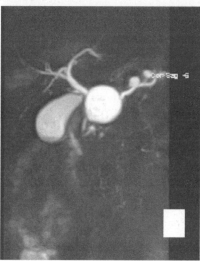

Fig. 3 Magnetic resonance cholangiopancreatography (MRCP) showing (A) a dilated pancreatic duct along its length with filling defects in the proximal duct and (B) a well-defined cystic lesion causing mass effect, and two further cystic lesions communicating with the main pancreatic duct representing side branch IPMN.

resonance cholangiopancreatography (MRCP; Fig. 3 & 4). Three-phase helical CT and dynamic MR imaging have been shown to be particularly useful in diagnosis.[15] The typical feature of IPMN is cystic dilatation of the main pancreatic duct and/or of the branch ducts; nodules and papillary projections, which are significantly associated with the presence of malignant neoplasms, usually appearing as filling defects within the cystic lesions. CT and MRCP can localise the tumour and assess its relationship with vessels and other organs. MRCP is particularly useful in the characterisation of single or multifocal branch duct IPMN, given its ability to demonstrate a communication between the main duct and the cyst.

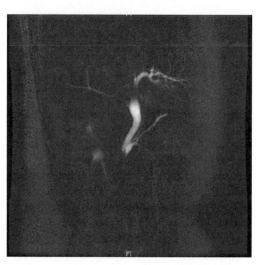

Fig. 4 Magnetic resonance cholangiopancreatogram (MRCP) with secretin showing a dilated parallel pancreatic head radical indicating a small branch duct IPMN.

Initial work-up of patients with suspected IPMN may also include contrast-enhanced ultrasonography, which is able to identify and characterise the 'cysts'. Endoscopic ultrasonography (Fig. 5 & 6) may be helpful in cases in which the diagnosis is uncertain. Endoscopic ultrasonography can study the main pancreatic duct, the presence of nodules or small projections in the main duct and / or in the cyst communicating with it. Moreover, endoscopic ultrasonography-guided fine needle aspiration may be done; fine needle aspiration can be obtained using transabdominal ultrasonography, which has the advantage of being less invasive. Cytological examination and detection of the K-ras mutation in pancreatic juice can indicate the presence of a malignant IPMN, even though this procedure has a low sensitivity (< 20%). The CEA level in pancreatic juice can be very useful in differentiating benign from malignant IPMNs. However, endoscopic ultrasonography with or without fine needle aspiration is considered to be a 'second level' procedure which should be done only in selected cases.

Cytological evaluation of pancreatic juice and subclassification (including immunochemical testing for MUC proteins), according to criteria previously described for histological diagnosis, have also been shown to be useful in pre-operative evaluation.[16] In recent years, intraductal endoscopy and / or peroral pancreatoscopy have been introduced. Experience is limited with these approaches and further studies are needed.

Evaluation with blood tests, including tumour markers, should be done in very case.

The diagnostic work-up of suspected IPMN aims to:

1. *Make the correct diagnosis of IPMN and differentiate it from other cystic neoplasms such as serous cystadenoma or mucinous cystic neoplasms or other cystic lesions of the pancreas (pseudocyst, true pancreatic cyst).*

2. *Differentiate between main-duct and branch-duct IPMN.*

3. *Identify those parameters which are associated with high risk of malignancy.*

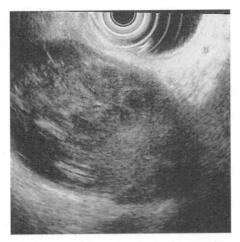

Fig. 5 Endoscopic ultrasound showing cystic dilatation of the pancreatic duct.

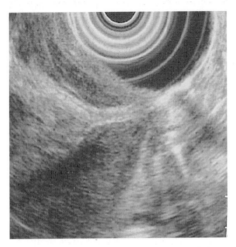

Fig. 6 Dilated common bile duct and pancreatic duct containing echogenic mucin.

The following parameters have been proven to be associated with malignancy in IPMNs: (i) presence of symptoms, particularly of jaundice, steatorrhea and new onset or worsening diabetes; (ii) diameter of the cystic lesion (> 30 mm); (iii) nodules, thick walls, papillary projections; (iv) dilated main pancreatic duct (> 10 mm); and (v) elevated CEA levels (> 120 ng/ml) in the pancreatic juice.

More recently, consensus indications for resection and scoring systems (incorporating such parameters as pancreatic duct size, jaundice and diabetes mellitus) have been proposed to predict the likelihood of finding malignancy in IPMN and to guide subsequent proposed management.[17–19]

NON-OPERATIVE MANAGEMENT

Recently, the International Association of Pancreatology proposed clear guidelines for the management of IPMNs. The guidelines state that all suspected main-duct and combined IPMNs should be resected, even in asymptomatic patients, since the risk of malignancy is high among these patients and there is no way to distinguish between benign and malignant IPMN pre-operatively. A recent, retrospective analysis in one centre of 60 resections for cystic pancreatic neoplasms supported an aggressive surgical approach to their management, given the difficulty in reliably distinguishing lesions pre-operatively.[20]

Branch-duct IPMN are associated with malignancy in about 25% of cases and patients with malignant branch-duct IPMN are more likely symptomatic, have a bigger lesion (> 3 cm) and have mural nodules.[2,9–11] Surgical resection is recommended in these cases, while asymptomatic patients with small (< 30 mm) branch-duct IPMN without nodules can be managed with careful observation.[2] It is important that this non-operative approach is carried out in experienced centres and data from large series are needed to validate this approach.[2]

A prospective study assessed the non-operative management of asymptomatic patients affected by a suspected branch-duct IPMN (evidence of a cystic lesion clearly communicating with a normal main pancreatic duct at MRCP) with a diameter less than 3.5 cm and without nodules, papillae, and with normal tumour markers.[21] In this study, ERCP and endoscopic ultrasonography were not routinely employed but were used only in those cases with an unclear diagnosis. The follow-up was carried out with contrast enhanced ultrasonography and MRCP every 6 months for the first 2 years and yearly thereafter. Between 2000 and 2003, 109 patients were observed. Twenty patients (18.3%) underwent immediate surgery because of the presence of symptoms and/or parameters associated with malignancy. Pathological diagnosis of branch-duct IPMN was confirmed in all and only two patients had an invasive carcinoma (10%), while one (5%) a carcinoma *in situ*. Eighty-nine patients (81.7%) were followed up for a median of 32 months; of these, 57 (64%) had multifocal disease. After a mean follow-up of 18.2 months, five patients (5.6%) showed an increase in the size of the lesion and underwent surgery. The pathological diagnosis was branch-duct adenoma in three patients and borderline in two.

This study suggests that in very well selected cases, a non-operative approach is safe and feasible and that the biological behaviour of branch-duct IPMNs is different if compared to those occurring in the main duct.

Key point 5

- Main-duct IPMN should be resected even in asymptomatic patients. Small branch-duct IPMN (< 30 mm) without mural nodules can be managed with careful observation in experienced centres.

SURGICAL MANAGEMENT

MAIN-DUCT IPMNS

The surgical management of main-duct IPMNs represents a challenge for the surgeon. Whilst in other pancreatic tumours, pre-operative studies can accurately locate the tumour and accordingly plan a pancreatic resection, this is not always the case in main-duct IPMN. In fact, pre-operative studies can show only a segmental dilatation of the main pancreatic duct with or without cysts. Dilatation may occur both proximally and distally to the tumour because of overproduction of mucus, making localisation of the neoplasm more problematic. Finally, main-duct IPMN can spread to involve the whole duct.

Typical resections include pancreaticoduodenectomy, left pancreatectomy, total pancreatectomy, according to the site and extension of the disease. Lymph node dissection must be performed as would be done for known invasive tumour, because of the high risk of invasion and the difficulty of pre-operative diagnosis. Limited resections, such as middle pancreatectomy, have been proposed for main-duct IPMN, but high rates of positive resection margins and recurrences when this procedure was performed for main-duct IPMN have been reported.[2,22,23] For these reasons, it is believed that standard resections should be performed in this condition.

Intra-operative examination of the transection margin is of paramount importance in the management of patients affected with main-duct IPMN.[2,5,24] Since IPMN may extend along the main pancreatic duct, it is important to assess the presence of tumour at the margin. Different outcomes are seen in groups with the surgical margin: 'negative' with normal epithelium in the main duct, 'de-epithelialised' with denuded epithelium or 'positive' for adenoma, or borderline or carcinoma.

> **Key point 6**
>
> • A typical resection should be performed according to the site and extent of the disease and extended if indicated after examination of the frozen section.

De-epithelialisation should not be considered as a negative margin since local recurrence can occur.[7] The presence of high-grade dysplasia or carcinoma requires an extension of the surgical resection up to total pancreatectomy; in cases of de-epithelialisation, adenoma or borderline tumour at the surgical margin, the optimal surgical strategy remains controversial:[2] extension of the resection a few centimetres to try to obtain a negative resection margin is one approach. Results from one centre show that, of 140 patients affected by main-duct IPMN who underwent surgical resection, the rate of negative margins in the surgical specimen was 58.5%, and the results of the intra-operative frozen section analysis modified the surgical plan, leading to an extension of the resection or to total pancreatectomy in 29 patients (20.7%).[5]

Recurrence in the pancreatic remnant may develop even if the transection margin is negative and even in patients with non-invasive disease.[8,9] Recurrence in the pancreatic remnant after resection of a main-duct IPMN can be due to three factors:

1. *The presence of a 'positive' resection margin.*

2. *Main-duct IPMN can be multicentric with synchronous 'skip' lesions along the main duct, still present at the time of surgery.*

3. *Given that IPMN may be a marker of a 'field defect' associated with a propensity for tumour development, metachronous lesions may occur years later in the remnant.*

For all these reasons, the role of total pancreatectomy in IPMN should be carefully evaluated and individualised. Some authors have reported that for malignant IPMN the frequency of recurrence (local recurrence or distant metastases) is similar whether or not total pancreatectomy was performed.[25,26] Chari *et al.*[9] reported a recurrence rate of 62% after total pancreatectomy and of 67% after partial pancreatectomy. The risks and long-term complications of total pancreatectomy must be considered and discussed with patients. A recent study (though limited by numbers) reported no recurrence at 127 months after pylorus preserving total pancreatectomy.[27] Finally, in patients with main-duct IPMN undergoing pylorus-preserving pancreaticoduodenectomy, pancreaticogastrostomy can be preferred instead of pancreaticojejunostomy. This may permit direct access by endoscopy to the pancreatic stump during follow-up, and allow direct opacification of the main pancreatic duct and sampling of pancreatic juice for cytological examination.[28,29]

BRANCH-DUCT IPMNS

A typical resection should be performed for branch-duct IPMNs. For asymptomatic patients with a small single lesion (< 3 cm) of the neck of the pancreas, without any suspicion of malignancy, a middle pancreatectomy can be considered.

In the case of multifocal disease, a total pancreatectomy or an extended standard resection would be necessary to assure radical treatment; however, a more selective approach can be considered with resection of the segment of the gland with the biggest or most suspicious lesion and close postoperative follow-up of the remnant. In multifocal branch-duct IPMNs, surgery must be performed in symptomatic patients and in those cases with radiological findings suggesting the presence of a malignant tumour.

Key points 7 & 8

- In branch-duct IPMNs, a typical resection should be performed when indicated.

- In cases of multifocal disease, a total pancreatectomy or an extended standard resection would be necessary to assure radical treatment.

Intra-operative frozen section is not usually performed for branch-duct IPMN. This might be done in the case of a malignant tumour, when an incomplete resection or involvement of the main pancreatic duct is suspected. At final histopathological examination, it is always important to rule out an extension of the IPMN from the branch duct system to the main pancreatic duct, since the biological behaviour of 'combined' main-duct–branch-duct IPMN seems to be similar to main-duct IPMN.

Key points 9 & 10

- In side-branch duct IPMNs, the value of intra-operative frozen section is not clear.

- Final histopathological examination should rule out an extension of the IPMN from the branch duct system to the main pancreatic duct.

FOLLOW-UP AND RE-RESECTION

After resection, strict follow-up should be adhered to. Patients affected by malignant IPMN are at higher risk of recurrence, but neoplastic recurrence can develop even in the presence of a benign tumour with negative resection margins, particularly in the case of main-duct IPMN. It is important to detect a 'recurrence' or development of new disease in the remnant since another resection should be considered in these cases.[2,7,8] In 140 resected patients affected by main-duct IPMN, eight (7%) developed a recurrence in the remnant.[5] Of these, seven had invasive carcinoma at initial histology while the remaining patient had an adenoma with negative resection margin; this patient underwent a completion pancreatectomy for a carcinoma *in situ*.

A clinical-laboratory-radiological evaluation can be conducted every 6 months in cases with malignant tumours and yearly for benign IPMNs. Radiological follow-up can include ultrasonography, CT or MRCP.

With regard to multifocal, branch-duct IPMN patients who underwent partial pancreatectomy, strict follow-up should be performed to evaluate the lesion or lesions in the remnant and possible development of new tumours. MRCP is particularly useful in this setting.[30]

Key points 11 & 12

- Patients with malignant main-duct IPMN are at high risk of recurrence; however, recurrence can develop even in benign IPMNs with negative resection margins.

- A close follow-up policy including ultrasonography, computed tomography or magnetic resonance cholangiopancreatography should be adopted.

PROGNOSIS

The survival of patients with IPMN can be good, even when the lesion is malignant and invasive. In recent experience with follow-up of 137 resected patients, 5- and 10-year disease-specific survival for 80 patients with adenoma, borderline and *in situ* carcinoma was 100% while for 57 patients with invasive carcinoma it was 60% and 50%, respectively.[5] In other large series, the 5-year disease-specific survival for IPMN with invasive carcinoma ranged from 36% to 43%.[8,9,25,31]

The rate of lymph node metastases in patients affected by malignant IPMN ranges from 16% to 46%.[5,7-9,25,32] In our experience, 41% of 58 patients with invasive main-duct IPMN had nodal metastases and had a 5-year survival rate of 45%, which was not significantly different to that of patients with invasive carcinoma and negative nodes.[5]

These observations suggest that adenocarcinoma arising in IPMN is probably a different disease entity when compared to ductal adenocarcinoma, in which long-term survival in patients with positive nodes is a rare event.

Key point 13

- Overall, the long-term survival for IPMN is very good in non-invasive tumours; however, the prognosis of IPMN even with invasive cancer is much better than that reported for ductal adenocarcinoma.

Key points for clinical practice

- The incidence of intraductal papillary mucinous neoplasms (IPMNs) has increased significantly in the last decade due to improvement in the radiological diagnosis and better understanding and correct classification of this disease.

- Main-duct IPMNs are more frequently associated with malignancy and invasive carcinoma. Differentiation between main- and branch-duct IPMNs is essential for correct clinical decision-making.

- Main-duct IPMNs are more likely to present with symptoms such as abdominal pain, pancreatitis, steatorrhea and, less commonly, jaundice, diabetes and weight loss.

- Branch-duct IPMNs can present with abdominal pain or pancreatitis. A large proportion of them, however, are asymptomatic and neoplasms are detected incidentally during radiological investigation of other systems.

- Main-duct IPMN should be resected even in asymptomatic patients. Small branch-duct IPMN (< 30 mm) without mural nodules can be managed with careful observation in experienced centres.

- A typical resection should be performed according to the site and extent of the disease and extended if indicated after examination of the frozen section.

- In branch-duct IPMNs, a typical resection should be performed when indicated.

- In cases of multifocal disease, a total pancreatectomy or an extended standard resection would be necessary to assure radical treatment.

- In side-branch duct IPMNs, the value of intra-operative frozen section is not clear.

- Final histopathological examination should rule out an extension of the IPMN from the branch duct system to the main pancreatic duct.

- Patients with malignant main-duct IPMN are at high risk of recurrence; however, recurrence can develop even in benign IPMNs with negative resection margins.

- A close follow-up policy including ultrasonography, computed tomography or magnetic resonance cholangiopancreatography should be adopted.

- Overall, the long-term survival for IPMN is very good in non-invasive tumours; however, the prognosis of IPMN even with invasive cancer is much better than that reported for ductal adenocarcinoma.

References

1. Carbognin G, Zamboni G, Pinali L et al. Branch duct IPMNs: value of cross-sectional imaging in the assessment of biological behavior and follow-up. *Abdom Imaging* 2006; **31**: 320–325.

2. Tanaka M, Chari S, Adsay V et al. International consensus guidelines for management of intraductal papillary mucinous neoplasms and mucinous cystic neoplasms of the pancreas. *Pancreatology* 2005; **6**: 17–32.

3. Ohashi K, Murakami Y, Murayama M, Takekoshi T, Ohta H, Ohashi I. Four cases of mucus secreting pancreatic cancer. *Prog Dig Endosc* 1982; **20**: 348–351.

4. Lim JH, Lee G, Oh YL. Radiologic spectrum of intraductal papillary mucinous tumor of the pancreas. *Radiographics* 2001; **21**: 323–340.

5. Salvia R, Fernandez-del Castillo C, Bassi C et al. Main-duct intraductal papillary mucinous neoplasms of the pancreas: clinical predictors of malignancy and long-term survival following resection. *Ann Surg* 2004; **239**: 678–685.

6. Wada K, Takada T, Yasuda H et al. Does 'clonal progression' relate to the development of intraductal papillary mucinous tumors of the pancreas? *J Gastrointest Surg* 2004; **8**: 289–296.

7. Falconi M, Salvia R, Bassi C, Zamboni G, Talamini G, Pederzoli P. Clinicopathological features and treatment of intraductal papillary mucinous tumour of the pancreas. *Br J Surg* 2001; **88**: 376–381.

8. Sohn TA, Yeo CJ, Cameron JL et al. Intraductal papillary mucinous neoplasms of the pancreas: an updated experience. *Ann Surg* 2004; **239**: 788–797.

9. Chari ST, Yadav D, Smyrk TC et al. Study of recurrence after surgical resection of intraductal papillary mucinous neoplasm of the pancreas. *Gastroenterology* 2002; **123**: 1500–1507.

10. Kobari M, Egawa S, Shibuya K et al. Intraductal papillary mucinous tumors of the pancreas comprise 2 clinical subtypes: differences in clinical characteristics and surgical management. *Arch Surg* 1999; **134**: 1131–1136.

11. Terris B, Ponsot P, Paye F et al. Intraductal papillary mucinous tumors of the pancreas confined to secondary ducts show less aggressive pathologic features as compared with those involving the main pancreatic duct. *Am J Surg Pathol* 2000; **24**: 1372–1377.

12. Sugiyama M, Izumisato Y, Abe N, Masaki T, Mori T, Atomi Y. Predictive factors for malignancy in intraductal papillary-mucinous tumours of the pancreas. *Br J Surg* 2003; **90**: 1244–1249.

13. Abu-Hilal M, Salvia R, Casaril A et al. Obstructive chronic pancreatitis and/or intraductal papillary mucinous neoplasms (IPMNs): a 21-year long case report. *JOP J Pancreas (Online)* 2006; **7**: 218–221.

14. Talamini G, Zamboni G, Salvia R et al. Intraductal papillary mucinous neoplasms and chronic pancreatitis. *Pancreatology* 2006; **6**: 626–634.

15. Yamada Y, Mori H, Matsumoto S. Intraductal papillary mucinous neoplasms of the pancreas: correlation of helical CT and dynamic MR imaging features with pathologic findings. *Abdom Imaging* 2007; E-pub ahead of print.

16. Hibi Y, Fukushima N, Tsuscida A et al. Pancreatic juice cytology and subclassification of intraductal papillary mucinous neoplasms of the pancreas. *Pancreas* 2007; **34**: 197–204.

17. Fujino Y, Matsumoto I, Ueda T, Toyama H, Juroda Y. Proposed new score predicting malignancy of intraductal papillary mucinous neoplasms of the pancreas. *Am J Surg* 2007; **194**: 304–307.

18. Pelaez-Luna M, Chari ST, Smyrk TC et al. Do consensus indications for resection in branch duct intraductal papillary mucinous neoplasm predict malignancy? A study of 147 patients. *Am J Gastroenterol* 2007; **102**: 1759–1764.

19. Murakami Y, Uemaura K, Hayashidani Y, Sudo T, Sueda T. Predictive factors of malignant or invasive intraductal papillary-mucinous neoplasms of the pancreas. *J Gastrointest Surg* 2007; **11**: 338–344.

20. Hardacre JM, McGee MF, Stellato TA, Schulak JA. An aggressive surgical approach is warranted in the management of cystic pancreatic neoplasms. *Am J Surg* 2007; **193**: 374–378.

21. Salvia R, Crippa S, Falconi M et al. Branch-duct intraductal papillary mucinous neoplasms of the pancreas: to operate or not to operate? *Gut* 2007; **56**: 1086–1090.

22. Sauvanet A, Partensky C, Sastre B *et al*. Medial pancreatectomy: a multi-institutional retrospective study of 53 patients by the French Pancreas Club. *Surgery* 2002; **132**: 836–843.

23. Crippa S, Bassi C, Warshaw AL *et al*. Middle pancreatectomy: indications, short- and long-term operative outcomes. *Ann Surg* 2007; **246**: 69–76.

24. Couvelard A, Sauvanet A, Kianmanesh R *et al*. Frozen sectioning of the pancreatic cut surface during resection of intraductal papillary mucinous neoplasms of the pancreas is useful and reliable. A prospective evaluation. *Ann Surg* 2005; **242**: 774–780.

25. Jang JY, Kim SW, Ahn YJ *et al*. Multicenter analysis of clinicopathologic features of intraductal papillary mucinous tumor of the pancreas: is it possible to predict the malignancy before surgery? *Ann Surg Oncol* 2005; **12**: 124–132.

26. Maire F, Hammel P, Terris B *et al*. Prognosis of malignant intraductal papillary mucinous tumours of the pancreas after surgical resection. Comparison with pancreatic ductal adenocarcinoma. *Gut* 2002; **51**: 717–722.

27. Inagaki M, Obara M, Kino S *et al*. Pylorus-preserving total pancreatectomy for an intraductal papillary-mucinous neoplasm of the pancreas. *J Hepatobiliary Pancreat Surg* 2007; **14**: 264–269.

28. Gigot JF, Deprez P, Sempoux C *et al*. Surgical management of intraductal papillary mucinous tumors of the pancreas: the role of routine frozen section of the surgical margin, intraoperative endoscopic staged biopsies of the Wirsung duct, and pancreaticogastric anastomosis. *Arch Surg* 2001; **136**: 1256–1262.

29. Bassi C, Butturini G, Salvia R, Crippa S, Falconi M, Pederzoli P. Open pancreatico-gastrostomy after pancreaticoduodenectomy: a pilot study. *J Gastrointest Surg* 2006; **10**: 1072–1080.

30. Pilleul F, Rochette A, Partensky C, Scoazec JY, Bernard P, Valette PJ. Preoperative evaluation of intraductal papillary mucinous tumors performed by pancreatic magnetic resonance imaging and correlated with surgical and histopathologic findings. *J Magn Reson Imaging* 2005; **21**: 237–244.

31. D'Angelica M, Brennan MF, Suriawinata AA, Klimstra D, Conlon KC. Intraductal papillary mucinous neoplasms of the pancreas. *Ann Surg* 2004; **239**: 400–408.

32. Wada K, Kozarek RA, Traverso LW. Outcomes following resection of invasive and noninvasive intraductal papillary mucinous neoplasms of the pancreas. *Am J Surg* 2005; **189**: 632–637.

Gary K. Atkin   Jeremy I. Livingstone

8

Gastrointestinal stromal tumours

Gastrointestinal stromal tumours (GISTs) are a type of neoplasm arising from the embryological mesoderm of the gastrointestinal tract. Originally, they were labelled as smooth muscle tumours, but it was clear that mesenchymal tumours of the gut were a distinct biological entity, as they had morphological and immunohistochemical features dissimilar to smooth muscle.[1] in addition, unlike sarcomas of the trunk or limbs, they were resistant to conventional chemotherapy agents.[2] The non-specific collective term 'gastrointestinal stromal tumour' was used initially to describe all gastrointestinal mesenchymal tumours.[3] However, it was clear the group had variable histological features and, in 1998, Hirota *et al.*[4] reported the association between GISTs and mutations of a receptor tyrosine kinase known as KIT. This allowed the separation of GISTs from other mesenchymal tumours based on their positive immunostaining for KIT, and led to the current classification of gastrointestinal mesenchymal tumours into GISTs, smooth muscle tumours, and neural tumours (schwannomas).

PATHOLOGY

GISTs are uncommon, comprising only 1–3% of all gastrointestinal neoplasia.[5] They are, however, the most common mesenchymal tumour of the gut.[6] They can occur at any age, but the peak age of presentation is 58 years.[1] They affect males and females equally,[7] and their true incidence is unknown, as a significant proportion are asymptomatic. Population-based studies estimate the incidence to be 15–20 per million for symptomatic tumours.[8]

Gary K. Atkin MRCS MD (for correspondence)
Specialist Registrar, Department of Upper Gastrointestinal Surgery, Watford General Hospital, Vicarage Road, Watford, Hertfordshire WD18 0HB, UK. E-mail: gkatkin@blueyonder.co.uk

Jeremy I. Livingstone FRCS MS
Consultant Surgeon, Department of Upper Gastrointestinal Surgery, Watford General Hospital, Vicarage Road, Watford, Hertfordshire WD18 0HB, UK.

Table 1 Site of origin of GISTs[1]

Site	Frequency
Oesophagus	5%
Stomach	50%
Small intestine	25%
Colon and rectum	10%
Extra-intestinal (mesentery, gallbladder, pancreas)	10%

GISTs may arise in any part of the gastrointestinal tract (Table 1), but are most commonly found in the stomach (Fig. 1). In the oesophagus, colon, and rectum, true smooth muscle tumours are more common.[2] Half the patients have metastatic disease at presentation, usually to the liver or peritoneum.[6] Lymph node involvement and extra-abdominal extension are very rare, occurring in less than 1% of cases.[1] This low risk of lymphatic spread has important implications on their surgical management. Median tumour size at presentation is 5 cm.[9] GISTs originate in the submucosal, muscular or serosal layers, and macroscopically they are unencapsulated and show cystic degeneration, necrosis or haemorrhage. They are often soft and fragile, necessitating careful handling during surgery to avoid tumour spillage.[10]

Histologically, there are three subtypes depending on the predominant cell type – spindle-shaped (70%), epithelioid (20%), or a combination of the two (10%).[11] The spindle cell tumours are often arranged in fascicles, whereas the epithelioid cells aggregate into nests. Pleomorphism is very rare, and mitotic

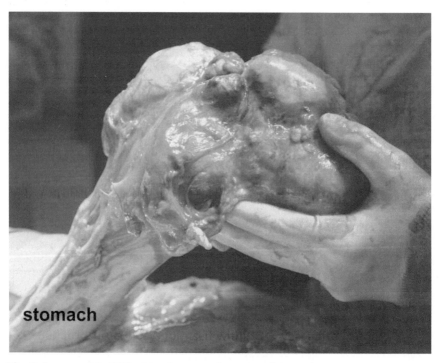

stomach

Fig. 1 Large gastric GIST arising from greater curve of stomach.

activity is minimal.[1] In 10–20% of tumours, there are characteristic hyaline or fibrillary structures known as skeinoid fibres.[12] Pathologically, their differential diagnosis includes true smooth muscle tumours (leiomyomas and leiomyosarcomas), schwannomas, inflammatory fibroid polyps and desmoid fibromatosis.[1] Gastrointestinal autonomic nerve tumours (GANTs) are a variant of GISTs in which there is a predominant neural differentiation.

IMMUNOHISTOCHEMICAL PROFILING

The defining feature of most GISTs is their positive immunohistochemical staining pattern for the receptor tyrosine kinase, KIT.[13] This is the product of the proto-oncogene *c-kit*, and is a transmembrane protein with an extracellular binding site for its ligand (stem cell factor; SCF) and an intracellular kinase site. Activation by SCF leads to the phosphorylation, and hence activation, of other intracellular signalling pathways, controlling cellular functions such as cell proliferation, chemotaxis, and apoptosis.[1] KIT is expressed in a number of cell types, but KIT mutations occurring in the interstitial cells of Cajal (ICC), the unique pacemaker cells that control peristalsis within the gut, have been shown to lead to GIST formation. Recent evidence suggests there are interstitial Cajal-like cells (ICLC) in extra-intestinal sites, and these are the presumed cell of origin for extra-intestinal GISTs.[14]

The KIT gene contains 21 exons, but mutations associated with GISTs have only been described in four – exons 9, 11, 13, and 17. Exon 11 mutations are the most common, and are found in 60–70% of GISTs.[4] KIT mutations are also implicated in the pathogenesis of other tumour types, such as seminomas and T-cell lymphomas; interestingly, these harbour mutations never seen in GISTs and very rarely contain mutations in exon 11 that are typical of GISTs.[1]

CD117 is an antibody to an epitope of KIT, and is the marker used to identify KIT-positive tumours. Some 95% of GISTs are positive for CD117 (Table 2),[11] whereas 60–70% of GISTs are positive for CD34 (a haematopoietic

Table 2 Immunohistochemical staining pattern of GISTs[11]

Marker	Frequency
CD117	95%
CD34	60–70%
Smooth muscle actin	30–40%
S-100	5%
Desmin	1–2%
Keratin	1–2%

Table 3 Differential staining features of gastrointestinal mesenchymal tumours[13]

	GISTs	Smooth muscle tumours	Neural tumours
CD117	95% +	–	–
CD34	60–70% +	10–15%	+
Smooth muscle actin	30–40% +	+	–
Desmin	Rare	+	–
S-100	5% +	Rare	+

progenitor cell antigen), and 30–40% are positive for smooth muscle actin. GISTs are rarely positive for S-100, a neural marker, or the muscle marker, desmin. This allows differentiation of GISTs from other mesenchymal tumours (Table 3). A few other tumour types are positive for KIT, including melanomas and germ cell tumours, but these rarely affect the gut.[2]

Recently, other markers have been described which may be more sensitive and specific than CD117 for the diagnosis of GISTs. DOG1, a cDNA encoding a protein of unknown function, and protein kinase C theta, a signalling molecule involved in T-cell activation, have both been shown to be strongly expressed in GISTs, and may have a future role in their diagnosis.[15,16]

Key points 1–3

- Gastrointestinal stromal tumours (GISTs) are a type of neoplasm arising from the embryological mesoderm of the gastrointestinal tract.

- GISTs can affect any part of the gastrointestinal tract, most frequently the stomach, and can occur in extra-intestinal sites, such as the mesentery and pancreas.

- GISTs are due to gain-of-function receptor tyrosine kinase (KIT) mutations in interstitial cells of Cajal, the gut's pacemaker cell.

ESTIMATING THE RISK OF AGGRESSIVE BEHAVIOUR

Due to their unpredictable nature, it is impossible to classify any individual GIST as definitely benign or malignant. The consensus now is that all GISTs have the potential for aggressive behaviour, and a scoring system to estimate the risk of aggressive behaviour has been proposed (Fig. 2), utilising the prognostic factors tumour size and mitotic count.[13] This is only an estimate, however, as small tumours with a low mitotic count may metastasise early.[1] Other proposed adverse prognostic factors include mucosal ulceration,[17] telomerase activity,[18] and tumour site, as small intestinal GISTs have a worse prognosis than gastric GISTs.[11]

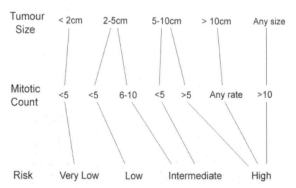

Fig. 2 Guidelines for prediction of aggressive behaviour of GISTs (mitotic count is per 50 high power fields).[13]

CLINICAL FEATURES

The clinical features of GISTs depend on their site of origin and are often non-specific, contributing to a delay in diagnosis. There may be symptoms due to the mass effect of the tumour (*e.g.* dysphagia with oesophageal GISTs), or secondary effects such as gastrointestinal haemorrhage and anaemia due to mucosal ulceration.[1] Non-specific symptoms such as abdominal pain, anorexia and weight loss are common with all GISTs, but particularly those in the stomach.[19] Colorectal lesions may present with rectal bleeding or change in bowel habit. Small tumours (< 2 cm) anywhere along the GI tract are usually asymptomatic and often detected incidentally.[2]

Other than occurring sporadically, it is now recognised that GISTs can also occur as part of several familial syndromes. The Carney Triad is the association of extra-adrenal paraganglioma, pulmonary chondroma, and gastric GISTs.[20] The majority of patients (85%) are women, and the condition usually presents before the age of 30 years, suggesting a germline mutation that is as yet undetermined. Of neurofibromastosis type 1 patients, 7% also develop GISTs.[21] These lesions tend to be multifocal with characteristic features, such as skeinoid fibres in 85% and positive S-100 staining in 60%.[22] Similarly, they rarely have mutations of KIT or PDGFRA.

DIAGNOSIS

The diagnosis of GISTs depends upon the tumour displaying the typical clinical, radiological, and pathological characteristics. Clinically, they occur along the GI tract or at certain extra-intestinal sites such as the mesentery, gallbladder, or pancreas. Pathologically, they must have the usual morphological and immunohistochemical features. Radiologically, they also display certain typical features. Contrast-enhanced CT is the imaging modality of choice for their diagnosis, as it is widely available and GISTs have a characteristic heterogeneous appearance, with central necrosis and areas of cystic degeneration (Fig. 3).[23] Endoscopic ultrasound may be a suitable alternative for small tumours and, as with adenocarcinoma, MRI is the modality of choice for rectal GISTs.[11] Controversy surrounds the use of

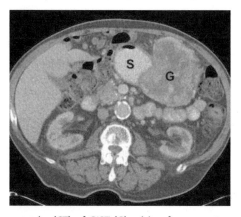

Fig. 3 Computed tomography (CT) of GIST (G) arising from greater curve of stomach (S) showing characteristic heterogeneous appearance.

percutaneous biopsy in the diagnosis of a suspected GIST due to the risk of tumour seeding; therefore, the initial diagnosis is often radiological with surgery providing definitive histology.[1] Occasionally, GISTs are encountered during emergency surgery for bowel obstruction or gastrointestinal bleeding. A GIST is suggested at laparotomy by a large mass without obvious lymph node involvement. The lesion should be resected *en-bloc*, and accurate histopathological assessment is needed to confirm the diagnosis and provide a risk of aggressive behaviour. Intra-abdominal open biopsy is discouraged due to the risk of tumour seeding, unless multiple metastatic lesions are already present.[11]

Key points 4–6

- All GISTs have the potential for aggressive behaviour, the risk being estimated from tumour size and mitotic count.

- The clinical features of GISTs depend on their site of origin and are often non-specific.

- Their diagnosis depends upon the tumour displaying the typical clinical, radiological, and pathological characteristics.

TREATMENT

Surgery remains the treatment of choice for operable disease. Recent advances in the non-surgical management of GISTs have improved the outcome for locally advanced and metastatic disease, and on-going investigation is aiming to determine the benefit of adjuvant therapy in resectable disease.

LOCALISED DISEASE

Surgery is the only effective treatment for localised disease and it is important for every patient with a GIST to be discussed at a multidisciplinary meeting so an experienced surgeon can determine tumour resectability.[11] The aim of surgery is to perform a curative resection whilst avoiding tumour spillage. A complete resection is associated with the best outcome,[6] and a non-curative resection should only be considered for palliation of symptoms such as bleeding or to reduce the mass effect of the tumour.[10] If resection margins are involved, re-excision is recommended provided the lesion does not involve the serosal surface.[11] Due to the rarity of lymphatic involvement, lymphadenectomy is not recommended unless there is obvious nodal disease at laparotomy.[11] Laparoscopy is also not recommended for most tumours due to the high risk of tumour rupture and seeding, but it might be appropriate for small (< 2 cm) intramural tumours particularly involving the stomach.[24]

Site-specific surgery

Oesophageal GISTs are rare and often require oesophagectomy because, as in the rectum and duodenum, limited surgical procedures may not be technically feasible.[11] Small gastric GISTs can be treated by limited wedge resections,[2] whereas larger tumours require subtotal or total gastrectomy (with or without omentectomy). Tumours affecting the small intestine are treated by segmental resection. Duodenal GISTs often occur in the second part, and so may require pancreaticoduodenectomy.[25] GISTs affecting the colorectum are treated as for carcinoma, with formal colectomy for colonic lesions, and anterior resection or abdominoperineal resection for rectal lesions.[25] Extra-intestinal GISTs should be resected *en bloc* with an adequate margin of normal tissue.[11]

Follow-up and management of recurrent disease following surgery

There are few data to guide the most appropriate strategy for follow-up after surgical resection, but a consensus statement suggests that for high- or intermediate-risk tumours follow-up by CT should be performed every 3–4 months for the first 3 years, then every 6 months until 5 years, then yearly thereafter [11]. For low or very low risk tumours, a CT should be performed every 6 months for 5 years. Recurrences following curative resections are predominantly intra-abdominal, and in particular hepatic, occurring at a median 20–25 months following the primary surgery.[8] Recurrent peritoneal disease should be treated by further resection whilst liver metastases are treated with adjuvant therapy.

IRRESECTABLE OR METASTATIC DISEASE

GISTs are not responsive to standard chemotherapy or radiotherapy,[26] and the median survival for irresectable or metastatic disease is 20 months.[7] Recently, the selective tyrosine kinase inhibitor imatinib mesylate has been shown to be effective in GIST patients. Known commercially as Glivec® (Novartis; Basel, Switzerland), it was originally developed for use in chronic myeloid leukaemia patients. Imatinib turns off the KIT intracellular signalling mechanism and so shifts the balance away from cellular proliferation towards apoptosis. It is given as an oral preparation, and has a long half-life, so it is usually administered once daily at a dose of 400 mg. It is well tolerated with few serious side-effects. Its efficacy has been confirmed in two phase III studies.[27,28] Recent 4-year follow-up data of a phase II study has demonstrated a median survival of 58 months with imatinib, compared with only 15 months for standard chemotherapy.[29]

The use of imatinib in resectable disease

Imatinib is currently only licensed for use in metastatic and irresectable GIST patients. It has not been compared against surgery for resectable disease and there is no evidence of benefit for its use following a curative resection. Its use as an adjuvant and neo-adjuvant agent is being investigated in on-going trials, but there is concern that it may actually reduce the efficacy of any subsequent course of treatment for recurrent disease or it may encourage the proliferation of imatinib-resistant clones. Currently, it may be considered for use in a neo-adjuvant setting when organ/function-sparing surgery is possible after treatment or when a metastasis may be rendered resectable following treatment.[11] Surgery should be performed after sufficient time to permit tumour shrinkage (usually 4–6 months).

Key points 7–8

- Surgery is the treatment of choice for localised disease.

- Irresectable or metastatic disease is best treated by drug therapy, the currently recommended agent being the tyrosine kinase inhibitor imatinib mesylate.

PROGNOSIS

The reported 5-year survival rate following a complete resection of a localised GIST is 48–70%, whereas for an incomplete resection it is 8–9%.[8,30] The median survival of patients with gastric GISTs is 39 months after a complete resection compared with 19 months following resection with a positive margin. Even with curative surgery for localised disease, reported recurrence rates are 40–80%, and long- term studies suggest that up to 90% of patients develop a recurrence or die from their disease.[8]

Key points for clinical practice

- Gastrointestinal stromal tumours (GISTs) are a type of neoplasm arising from the embryological mesoderm of the gastrointestinal tract.

- GISTs can affect any part of the gastrointestinal tract, most frequently the stomach, and can occur in extra-intestinal sites, such as the mesentery and pancreas.

- GISTs are due to gain-of-function receptor tyrosine kinase (KIT) mutations in interstitial cells of Cajal, the gut's pacemaker cell.

- All GISTs have the potential for aggressive behaviour, the risk being estimated from tumour size and mitotic count.

- The clinical features of GISTs depend on their site of origin and are often non-specific.

- Their diagnosis depends upon the tumour displaying the typical clinical, radiological, and pathological characteristics.

- Surgery is the treatment of choice for localised disease.

- Irresectable or metastatic disease is best treated by drug therapy, the currently recommended agent being the tyrosine kinase inhibitor imatinib mesylate.

References

1. Rubin BP. Gastrointestinal stromal tumours: an update. *Histopathology* 2006; **48**: 83–96.
2. Connolly EM, Gaffney E, Reynolds JV. Gastrointestinal stromal tumours. *Br J Surg* 2003; **90**: 1178–1186.

3. Mazur MT, Clark HB. Gastric stromal tumors. Reappraisal of histogenesis. *Am J Surg Pathol* 1983; **7**: 507–519.

4. Hirota S, Isozaki K, Moriyama Y *et al*. Gain-of-function mutations of *c-kit* in human gastrointestinal stromal tumors. *Science* 1998; **279**: 577–580.

5. Rossi CR, Mocellin S, Mencarelli R *et al*. Gastrointestinal stromal tumors: from a surgical to a molecular approach. *Int J Cancer* 2003; **107**: 171–176.

6. DeMatteo RP, Lewis JJ, Leung D *et al*. Two hundred gastrointestinal stromal tumors: recurrence patterns and prognostic factors for survival. *Ann Surg* 2000; **231**: 51–58.

7. Graadt van Roggen JF, van Velthuysen ML, Hogendoorn PC. The histopathological differential diagnosis of gastrointestinal stromal tumours. *J Clin Pathol* 2001; **54**: 96–102.

8. Eisenberg BL, Judson I. Surgery and imatinib in the management of GIST: emerging approaches to adjuvant and neoadjuvant therapy. *Ann Surg Oncol* 2004; **11**: 465–475.

9. Hasegawa T, Matsuno Y, Shimoda T, Hirohashi S. Gastrointestinal stromal tumor: consistent CD117 immunostaining for diagnosis, and prognostic classification based on tumor size and MIB-1 grade. *Hum Pathol* 2002; **33**: 669–676.

10. Roberts PJ, Eisenberg B. Clinical presentation of gastrointestinal stromal tumors and treatment of operable disease. *Eur J Cancer* 2002; **38 (Suppl 5)**: S37–S38.

11. Blay JY, Bonvalot S, Casali P *et al*. Consensus meeting for the management of gastrointestinal stromal tumors. Report of the GIST Consensus Conference of 20–21 March 2004, under the auspices of ESMO. *Ann Oncol* 2005; **16**: 566–578.

12. Plaat BE, Hollema H, Molenaar WM *et al*. Soft tissue leiomyosarcomas and malignant gastrointestinal stromal tumors: differences in clinical outcome and expression of multidrug resistance proteins. *J Clin Oncol* 2000; **18**: 3211–3220.

13. Fletcher CD, Berman JJ, Corless C *et al*. Diagnosis of gastrointestinal stromal tumors: a consensus approach. *Hum Pathol* 2002; **33**: 459–465.

14. Min KW, Leabu M. Interstitial cells of Cajal (ICC) and gastrointestinal stromal tumor (GIST): facts, speculations, and myths. *J Cell Mol Med* 2006; **10**: 995–1013.

15. West RB, Corless CL, Chen X *et al*. The novel marker, DOG1, is expressed ubiquitously in gastrointestinal stromal tumors irrespective of KIT or PDGFRA mutation status. *Am J Pathol* 2004; **165**: 107–113.

16. Blay P, Astudillo A, Buesa JM *et al*. Protein kinase C theta is highly expressed in gastrointestinal stromal tumors but not in other mesenchymal neoplasias. *Clin Cancer Res* 2004; **10**: 4089–4095.

17. Miettinen M, El-Rifai W, Lasota J. Evaluation of malignancy and prognosis of gastrointestinal stromal tumors: a review. *Hum Pathol* 2002; **33**: 478–483.

18. Kawai J, Kodera Y, Fujiwara M *et al*. Telomerase activity as prognostic factor in gastrointestinal stromal tumors of the stomach. *Hepatogastroenterology* 2005; **52**: 959–964.

19. D'Amato G, Steinert DM, McAuliffe JC, Trent JC. Update on the biology and therapy of gastrointestinal stromal tumors. *Cancer Control* 2005; **12**: 44–56.

20. Carney JA, Sheps SG, Go VL, Gordon H. The triad of gastric leiomyosarcoma, functioning extra-adrenal paraganglioma and pulmonary chondroma. *N Engl J Med* 1977; **296**: 1517–1518.

21. Zoller ME, Rembeck B, Oden A, Samuelsson M, Angervall L. Malignant and benign tumors in patients with neurofibromatosis type 1 in a defined Swedish population. *Cancer* 1997; **79**: 2125–2131.

22. Takazawa Y, Sakurai S, Sakuma Y *et al*. Gastrointestinal stromal tumors of neurofibromatosis type I (von Recklinghausen's disease). *Am J Surg Pathol* 2005; **29**: 755–763.

23. King DM. The radiology of gastrointestinal stromal tumours (GIST). *Cancer Imaging* 2005; **5**: 150–156.

24. Walsh RM, Ponsky J, Brody F, Matthews BD, Heniford BT. Combined endoscopic/laparoscopic intragastric resection of gastric stromal tumors. *J Gastrointest Surg* 2003; **7**: 386–392.

25. Berman J, O'Leary TJ. Gastrointestinal stromal tumor workshop. *Hum Pathol* 2001; **32**: 578–582.

26. Demetri GD. Identification and treatment of chemoresistant inoperable or metastatic GIST: experience with the selective tyrosine kinase inhibitor imatinib mesylate (STI571). *Eur J Cancer* 2002; **38 (Suppl 5)**: S52–S59.

27. Verweij J, Casali PG, Zalcberg J *et al.* Early efficacy comparison of two doses of imatinib for the treatment of advanced gastro-intestinal stromal tumors (GIST): interim results of a randomized phase III trial from the EORTC-STBSG, ISG and Agastrointestinal tractG. *Proc Am Soc Clin Oncol* 2003; **22**: A3272.

28. Rankin C, Von Mehren M, Blanke C *et al.* Dose effect of imatinib (IM) in patients (pts) with metastatic GIST – Phase III Sarcoma Group Study S0033. *J Clin Oncol* 2004; **22 (Suppl 14)**: A9005.

29. Blanke CD, Demetri GD, Von Mehren M *et al.* Long-term follow-up of a phase II randomized trial in advanced gastrointestinal stromal tumor (GIST) patients (pts) treated with imatinib mesylate. *J Clin Oncol* 2006; **24 (Suppl 18S)**: 9528.

30. Bucher P, Villiger P, Egger JF, Buhler LH, Morel P. Management of gastrointestinal stromal tumors: from diagnosis to treatment. *Swiss Med Wkly* 2004; **134**: 145–153.

Alistair F. Myers Tim J.C. Bryant
Nicholas E. Beck

9

Imaging the small bowel: new techniques and problems in clinical practice

The small bowel is difficult to investigate. With a median length of 5.7 m (range, 3.35–7.85 m),[1] it is made more difficult to visualise by location and anatomy. Investigations must traverse proximal or distal gut, and then negotiate a tortuous course. Even at laparotomy, mucosal detail may not easily be seen. The varied reasons for investigation (Table 1) require a range of imaging techniques. Barium contrast studies (small bowel follow-through, and small bowel enema (also known as enteroclysis) are still widely used although

Table 1 Common indications for small bowel investigation

- Investigation of non-specific symptoms such as pain, distension, bloating, diarrhoea
- Suspected inflammatory bowel disease, including exclusion of small bowel disease in Crohn's colitis
- Intermittent or partial small bowel obstruction
- Obscure GI bleeding, iron-deficient anaemia or bleeding per rectum with normal oesophagogastroduodenoscopy and colonoscopy
- Definition of anatomy, of fistulas or malrotation
- Exclusion of malignancy, for example, complicating coeliac disease

Alistair F. Myers MSc MRCS (for correspondence)
Specialist Registrar in Colorectal Surgery, Department of Surgery, Southampton General Hospital, Tremona Road, Southampton SO16 6YD, UK
E-mail: alistairmyers@hotmail.com

Tim J.C. Bryant BMedSci MRCP FRCR
Fellow in Interventional Radiology, Department of Radiology, Southampton General Hospital, Tremona Road, Southampton SO16 6YD, UK

Nicholas E. Beck PhD FRCS
Consultant Colorectal Surgeon, Department of Surgery, Southampton General Hospital, Tremona Road, Southampton SO16 6YD, UK

Table 2 Problems with studying the small bowel

- Location, *i.e.* the need to negotiate the upper or lower GI tracts first
- Movement, with consequent artefact
- Radiation dose
- Patient acceptability of, for example, nasogastric tubes, MRI scanners
- Low yield, arising from large volume, non-targeted, or inappropriate referrals
- Interpretation of images, *i.e.* do they explain the symptoms?

there are now many alternative small bowel imaging techniques. These include ultrasonography, computed tomography (CT) enteroclysis, CT enterography, magnetic resonance (MR) enteroclysis, (wireless) capsule endoscopy and enteroscopy. Enteroscopy includes push enteroscopy, push-pull (or double-balloon) enteroscopy and intra-operative enteroscopy. This range of choices helps to counter the difficulties listed in Table 2.

The relative yield of positive results for each study is partly established. Studies quote sensitivity and specificity but many have little follow-up data. At present, there is no definite gold standard reference. To be absolutely accurate would require corresponding histopathology from surgical resection or post-mortem examination, but this is rarely available. The supporting evidence is more often a combination of other investigations, such as endoscopy or cross-sectional imaging, histopathology from biopsy and clinical follow-up.

The comparison of studies into yield in suspected inflammatory bowel disease or Crohn's disease is made difficult by the varying definition of suspected Crohn's disease. The rarity of some small bowel diseases (*e.g.* primary malignancy) makes it difficult for any researcher to gain sufficient numbers to draw conclusions. In some indications, however, the usefulness of tests is better known. In gastrointestinal bleeding, approximately 95% of cases will be diagnosed by barium study or endoscopy of the upper or lower GI tracts. The remaining 5% will be arising from the small bowel.[2] Obscure GI bleeding is the term for the situation where oesophagogastroduodenoscopy (OGD) and colonoscopy do not show the source of bleeding. Small bowel enema has long been used to investigate this with varying results. Of 128 patients studied by Moch *et al.*,[3] 27 (21%) had confirmed or highly probable lesions found at enteroclysis, although yields in other series are often lower.

Key point 1

- The small bowel is difficult to image and studies of all techniques are limited by the lack of a gold standard reference and agreed criteria for referral.

BARIUM CONTRAST STUDIES

Small bowel contrast studies (*i.e.* small bowel follow-through and small bowel enema or enteroclysis) have been used for decades. Small bowel follow-through

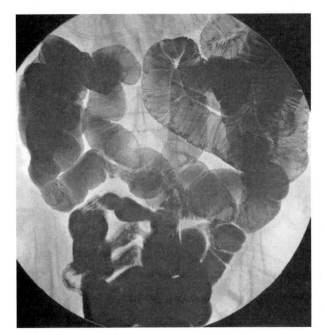

Fig. 1 Normal small bowel enema.

consists of a patient being given a barium suspension to drink along with an oral prokinetic such as metoclopramide (Fig. 1). The patient is laid prone and plain radiographs are taken periodically until the contrast reaches the caecum, with targeted fluoroscopy of specific areas of interest. Manual palpation of the abdomen facilitates movement of contrast and assessment of fixation of bowel loops. The advantages include the relative ease of the concept and its execution, the availability of equipment and expertise, the acceptance to the patient, and a relatively lower radiation dose. The disadvantages of the technique relate to the limited ability to distinguish abnormality, given that there may be many overlying loops of small intestine.[4] The consensus has long been in favour of small bowel enema being a superior technique.[4,5] This involves insertion of a nasojejunal tube through which the contrast medium is infused, followed by large volumes of methylcellulose or air to achieve double contrast. This technique produces marked distension of the lumen and demonstrates mucosal detail more readily. However, there is greater discomfort to the patient, a higher radiation dose and the possibility that gastroduodenal disease may not be seen. The investigation requires more experienced radiologists. Although many consider small bowel enema to be the superior test, specifically in the diagnosis of Crohn's disease[5] and other small bowel pathology (notably obstruction), this opinion is not universally held. Some radiologists advocate that small bowel follow-through with careful fluoroscopy and vigorous manual palpation can produce acceptable results with less cost, radiation exposure and discomfort to the patient (Fig. 2).[6–8]

The sensitivity and specificity of these contrast studies vary in the range of approximately 85–95% and 89–94%, respectively.[7,9] One large retrospective review of 1465 studies over 10 years rates claimed sensitivity of 93.1% and specificity of 96.7%, but diagnostic accuracy at 67.5%.[10] Follow-up was at least 5 years and findings were compared with clinical course and, where available, surgical findings (Fig. 3).

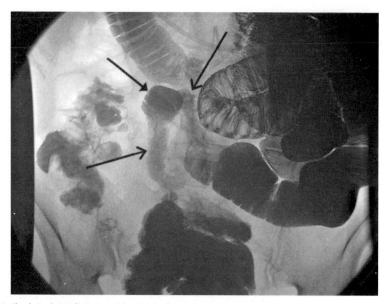

Fig. 2 Ileal Crohn's disease with skip lesions demonstrating mucosal oedema, cobble-stoning and ulceration (open arrows) with normal bowel in between (closed arrow).

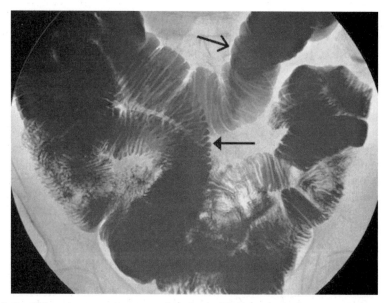

Fig. 3 Small bowel enema demonstrating classical fold reversal of untreated coeliac disease with ileal jejunisation (closed arrow) and reduction of normal jejunal fold frequency (open arrow).

Key point 2

- Barium contrast studies are widely available but yield is low.

ULTRASONOGRAPHY

Transabdominal ultrasound has been used to evaluate the small intestine, as it is cheap, quick, acceptable to patients and does not use ionising radiation. This is important as the radiation dose to Crohn's disease patients should be limited given the potential for many investigations over a life-time. However, its use has been limited by a lack of standardisation and the very observer-dependent nature of the test.[11] Studies tend to concentrate on the usefulness of ultrasonography in Crohn's disease specifically, with bowel wall thickening and the presence of mesenteric fat wrapping being used as markers of disease activity. Other signs include the pattern of vascularisation, the presence of free peritoneal fluid and mesenteric lymphadenopathy. Ultrasonography can also give direct extraluminal information, such as the presence of abscesses, which is missed or only indirectly inferred by small bowel contrast studies. It is postulated that similar changes may be seen in coeliac disease. It may be possible to look for lymphomas,[12] but this role is not well-defined (Fig.4).

Ultrasound remains particularly popular with paediatricians in view of the lack of harmful radiation and relative acceptability to the patient group, especially if many investigations will be required starting at a young age. Images are also better as children tend to have less body fat. A recent trial compared ultrasonography with small bowel follow-through and colonoscopy in a prospectively recruited cohort of 44 children.[13] When compared with small bowel follow-through of the ileum, ileal bowel wall thickening of > 2.5 mm gave comparative sensitivity of 75%, specificity of 92% and positive predictive value of 88%. Below 2.5 mm, however, the researchers concluded that even severe mucosal lesions could not be excluded. Superior mesenteric artery

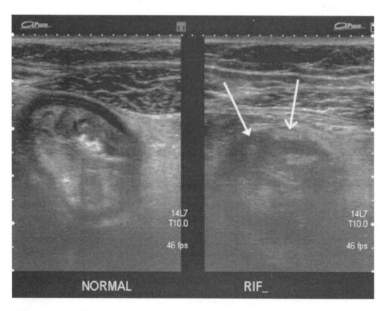

Fig. 4 Ultrasonography comparing normal and abnormal small bowel. Note the encroachment of the echogenic mesenteric fat onto the antimesenteric border, or 'fat wrapping' (open arrow), and loss of mural definition (closed arrow) consistent with active Crohn's disease.

Doppler did not correlate with disease severity. Previous studies have concluded that ultrasonography has a good positive predictive value in distal ileal Crohn's disease but that small bowel follow-through is more sensitive and is still indicated if there are strong clinical grounds in spite of a normal ultrasonography result.[14]

A recent meta-analysis of the role of ultrasonography in the detection of Crohn's disease has been published.[15] Two case-control studies and five cohort series fulfil criteria, having been performed on patients with clinical and/or laboratory data consistent with Crohn's disease. These compare ultrasound in the diagnosis of Crohn's disease with given reference standards. Because of the heterogeneity of values, pooled sensitivity and specificity data could not be calculated exactly, but was reported as being 75–94% and 67–100%, respectively. Furthermore, if a cut off for bowel wall thickness of > 3 mm was used, sensitivity of 88% and specificity of 93% were achieved and, if > 4 mm was used, these figures were 74% and 97%, respectively.

The limitations of ultrasound (Table 3) currently include the lack of agreed definitions of the level of bowel wall thickening that may be considered abnormal. Bowel wall thickening may be caused by other processes, such as ileal tuberculosis and the backwash ileitis of ulcerative colitis. It is not certain how different findings might be used in staging of known disease, gauging response to treatment as opposed to diagnosis.

Other developments may include supplementation with oral intestinal contrast. Calabrese *et al.*[16] compared standard transabdominal ultrasonography and ultrasonography after distension of the small bowel with an iso-osmolar polyethylene glycol electrolyte-balanced solution using small bowel enema as gold standard in 28 patients with known Crohn's disease. Correlation with small bowel enema was superior in the group which had received contrast ($r = 0.88$ versus $r = 0.64$ for the non-enhanced ultrasound), with greater lengths of diseased bowel being recognised and detection of jejunal lesions otherwise missed with plain ultrasonography. Pareante *et al.*[17] used a cheap and widely available non-absorbable anechoic contrast to distend the small bowel to improve visualisation in 102 consecutive patients with proven Crohn's disease. Sensitivity in detecting lesions was 91.4% for conventional ultrasound and 96.1% for post-contrast ultrasonography, with only one false negative in the

Table 3 Advantages and disadvantages of transabdominal ultrasound

Advantages
- Cheap
- Quick
- Patient acceptability
- No ionising radiation
- Extraluminal information
- Dynamic images

Disadvantages
- Highly observer-dependent
- Not widely available
- Less useful in the obese or in the presence of large volumes of bowel gas

contrast group. Strictures were also better seen. The authors concluded that ultrasonography with this contrast is comparable with small bowel enema and, therefore, could be a first-line investigation. Colour flow and Doppler ultrasonography evaluate the changes seen in vasculature with bowel inflammation. Increased vascularity is seen in the bowel wall. The superior mesenteric artery imaged using Doppler ultrasonography may indicate disease activity. Changes in flow variables, such as mean superior mesenteric artery diameter, resistive index and flow volume are considered to correlate with disease activity,[18] although other variables may not be reliable in clinical practice.[19] Only studies with small numbers are found in the literature and therefore the role of Doppler ultrasonography is still to be established.

Key point 3

- Ultrasonography may be very useful and acceptable in identifying terminal ileitis, particularly in children, but its use is very observer-dependent and expertise in bowel ultrasound is not widely available.

COMPUTED TOMOGRAPHY

CT has a central role in the investigation of the abdomen. It is widely available, quick, acceptable to most patients, relatively cheap and has the major advantage over luminal contrast studies that it provides additional extraluminal information (Table 4). CT can also depict bowel wall thickening, fistulas, abscesses and lymphadenopathy, and findings are not restricted to the small bowel.[9] Bowel wall enhancement during different phases of scanning with intravenous contrast allows assessment of perfusion. Intramural gas may be detected, especially with newer scanners. The advent of multidetector CT allows rapid acquisition of data sets with almost isotropic voxels allowing multiplanar reformatting. Thus, the data may be reconstructed to give images arranged at any angle. CT is often quicker and more easily available than MR.

The limitations of small bowel imaging with CT include the inherent risks of ionising radiation, the fact that it is a static rather than dynamic investigation (which may make differentiation between skip lesions and peristalsis difficult), and the artefact which may arise from the lack of physiological distension.

Table 4 Advantages and disadvantages of CT enteroclysis and enterography

Advantages
    Widely available
    Extraluminal information
    Reformatting possibilities
    Quick to perform

Disadvantages
    Ionising radiation
    Static images

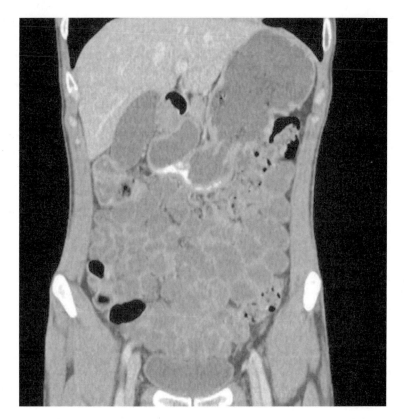

Fig. 5 Coronally-reformatted image obtained at CT enterography using negative oral contrast demonstrating normal small bowel.

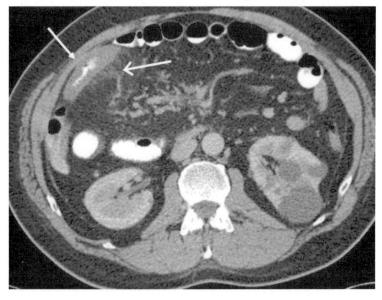

Fig. 6 Short segment terminal ileal Crohn's disease (closed arrow) with associated hazy inflammatory change in the mesenteric fat (open arrow).

CT enteroclysis is a newer, more specific small bowel technique requiring the same nasojejunal intubation and small bowel distension with contrast as barium enteroclysis. The images are gathered more quickly than those gathered at small bowel enema; however, the ability to follow the progression of contrast is lacking. Published data are limited to case reports or series. Although small numbers are reported and there is limited clinical follow-up, good results have been shown. In a comparison of CT enteroclysis and ileoscopy in 39 patients, of whom 30 had abnormal endoscopic findings, overall sensitivity and specificity of CT enteroclysis for ileal Crohn's disease detection were 86.7% and 100% (positive predictive value 100%, negative predictive value 69.2%).[20] The authors conclude that CT enteroclysis is as good as MR enteroclysis in the known Crohn's disease patient, and has the advantage of being cheaper, more acceptable to the patient and more readily available.

A prospective study of CT enteroclysis in 107 consecutive patients with wide indications for referral including suspected malignancy ($n = 8$), known inflammatory bowel disease ($n = 18$), occult GI bleeding ($n = 36$), low-grade small bowel obstruction ($n = 31$) and refractory coeliac sprue ($n = 14$), compared results with chosen supplementary imaging.[21] The authors reported the procedure being well-tolerated by all but one patient, which is somewhat lower than literature review would lead one to expect. Overall, true positive findings were found in 44 (41%) of patients, and true negative in 60 (56%) patients. Sensitivity was calculated as 100% and specificity 95%, positive predictive value 94% and negative predictive value 100%. In 17 patients, small bowel disease was only identified on CT enteroclysis. Of those with small bowel neoplasia (21), 9 were not seen on small bowel follow-through. These results are consistent with other series where, in 17 patients who underwent both CT enteroclysis and small bowel follow-through, tumours were missed or incomplete in 12 cases.[22] In the 31 cases of suspected low-grade obstruction, CT enteroclysis demonstrated all 12 cases where small bowel obstruction was found to be present, with the comment that this was missed by small bowel follow-through in 4 patients. With regard to Crohn's disease, appearances were comparable with small bowel follow-through in 9 patients, but CT enteroclysis demonstrated a fistula in three patients which was not shown on other modalities. In addition, CT enteroclysis was reported to aid in the diagnosis of ileocaecal tuberculosis in two patients by demonstrating necrotic mesenteric lymph nodes. Of those 14 patients with refractory coeliac sprue, CT enteroclysis demonstrated ulceration in three patients, lymphoma in two patients and adenocarcinoma of the jejunum in one patient. Although these numbers were small, the authors commented that the trend was in favour of CT enteroclysis, or at least that CT enteroclysis was no worse than small bowel enema.

Other studies have compared CT enteroclysis with small bowel contrast studies, with mixed results. Minordi et al.[23] compared small bowel enema with CT enteroclysis in 52 patients suspected of having small bowel disease. Of these, 30 would eventually be diagnosed with Crohn's disease, two with lymphoma, two with carcinoid and one with adhesions. Reporting a sensitivity of 83%, a specificity of 100% and a diagnostic accuracy of 89%, the authors concluded that CT enteroclysis was an effective technique overall but, importantly, that early Crohn's disease may be better demonstrated on small bowel enema as it was missed in five cases by CT enteroclysis. They also suggested that, in patients with a very high index of suspicion, use of both tests may be appropriate, if one did not provide an answer. Concerning Crohn's disease in particular, CT enteroclysis and small bowel enema were compared in 50 consecutive patients by Sailer et al.,[24] who also considered other follow-up data such as surgical findings and clinical course. Significantly more abnormalities in the small bowel were found with CT enteroclysis than small bowel enema ($P < 0.01$), but principally with the extraluminal manifestations.

CT enterography is a generic term for a CT investigation where the small bowel is distended with orally-ingested contrast as opposed to that delivered by nasojejunal tube in enteroclysis. The primary reason for abandoning the nasojejunal tube is patient acceptability; therefore, enterography must prove itself as effective as enteroclysis. Oral contrast agents tried include water, methylcellulose, dilute barium solution and polyethylene glycol (PEG) solution. A large series of clinical experience is emerging in the literature[25] and sensitivity is quoted in the range of 77–92%. Large comparative trials are awaited. Mazzeo et al.[26] have reported a retrospective series of 106 patients with CT enterography using PEG solution, compared with a variety of other assessments of the small bowel including endoscopy (45 patients), small bowel follow-through (55 patients) and surgery (28 patients). Overall sensitivity was 91%, specificity of 93% and accuracy 92%. There were five false-negative cases. Therefore, the advantage of oral hyperhydration to achieve small bowel distensibility is that in future it could be added to the general CT abdomen/pelvis examination being performed to investigate abdominal pain of uncertain aetiology.

Key point 4

- Computed tomography enteroclysis should be at least as good as small bowel enema, and will provide extraluminal information. Images are static and repeated studies, such as Crohn's patients might expect during a life-time, may result in considerable exposure to ionising radiation.

MAGNETIC RESONANCE IMAGING

MR has an increasing use in small bowel disease and Crohn's disease in particular. It has the advantages of CT in giving extraluminal information and permits multiplanar reformatting without ionising radiation (Table 5). This makes it especially preferable in children and those of reproductive age who may require repeat imaging over many years. The ability of MR to distinguish inflammation makes it particularly useful in Crohn's disease, as strictures caused by active disease may appear brighter on T2-weighted images than those caused by fibrosis.[27] Definition of tissue planes is better than on CT, although advances in CT and MR have tended to leap-frog over each other in recent years. Real-time functional information may be obtained with MR fluoroscopy and this is a distinct advantage over CT.

Table 5 Advantages and disadvantages of MR enteroclysis

Advantages
- Extraluminal information
- Reformatting possibilities
- Lack of ionising radiation
- Dynamic imaging
- Ability to differentiate layers of the bowel wall

Disadvantages
- Patient compliance
- Long scan acquisition times/artefact
- High cost
- Limited availability of scanning time

Luminal contrast may be provided by physiological luminal content or with purposeful distension, either by drinking or by enteroclysis. Positive gadolinium-based and negative iron-based contrast agents have been used in MR enteroclysis.[28] Bowel wall enhancement with a gadolinium-based contrast agent is useful in the assessment of inflammation and inflammatory bowel disease in particular. Using the widely available methylcellulose solution intraluminally creates good contrast between wall and lumen. Methylcellulose produces low-signal intensity on T1-weighted images and high-signal intensity on T2-weighted images, making it a useful biphasic contrast agent. MR has been shown to demonstrate the full spectrum of Crohn's disease manifestations, including mural ulcers, fistulas, pseudopolyps, thickening, stenosis and pre-stenotic dilatation (Fig. 7).[29]

The principal disadvantage of MR is patient compliance, with many patients failing to complete scans. Long acquisition times add to this, and may

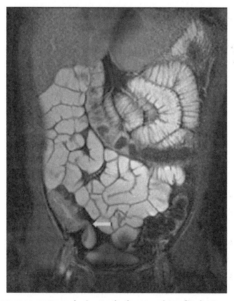

Fig. 7 Magnetic resonance enteroclysis study (coronal trufisp). Arrow indicates Crohn's disease terminal ileitis with stricture.

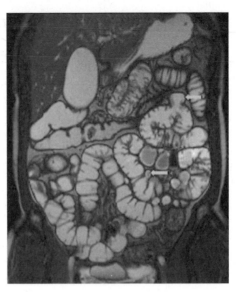

Fig. 8 Jejunal diverticulosis seen on magnetic resonance enteroclysis (coronal trufisp).

affect image quality, as artefact may be produced by peristalsis. Vomiting and inadvertent rectal evacuation also count against MR enteroclysis. Whilst rectal evacuation is undesirable, vomiting inside an MR scanner may be positively harmful, especially if sedation has been administered either for patient comfort and/or nasojejunal tube insertion.

MR and CT have been compared in various studies. MR was considered superior to single-phase helical CT scanning in a study of 26 patients,[30] showing significantly more abnormal segments of bowel. However, CT in the absence of luminal distension is not particularly sensitive for excluding small bowel pathology, and single-phase scanning is increasingly rare in the UK (Fig. 8).

Wiardia *et al.*[31] described a yield of 29 abnormal findings in 50 patients (58%) with close correlation between clinical course and study findings in 49 of 50 (98%). Comparative studies are also increasingly common in the literature. Masselli *et al.*[32] claimed the largest series in the literature comparing small bowel enema and MR enteroclysis, with 66 consecutive patients with known Crohn's disease. Lesions were seen in 44 patients on small bowel enema and 40 with MR enteroclysis, as recognised by experienced abdominal radiologists blinded to the outcome of the other study. There were no significant differences in findings of mural ulceration, pseudopolyps, stenosis, pre-stenotic dilatation or fistulas. There were significantly more extraluminal complications of Crohn's disease found with MR enteroclysis. These included abscesses, lymphadenopathy, small bowel separation and colonic lesions. If no more small bowel disease is found with MR enteroclysis than with small bowel enema, it makes it difficult to justify the use of a limited and expensive resource, as extraluminal information may be collated if required with other, cheaper and more available tests such as CT and ultrasonography. Other studies have compared MR enteroclysis with conventional small bowel enema, and have concluded that MR enteroclysis may be inferior in detecting subtle lesions.[33]

> **Key point 5**
>
> - MR enteroclysis may be equivalent to other imaging modalities, but with the advantage of dynamic imaging and no ionising radiation.

ENTEROSCOPY

Enteroscopy is an important field as it allows both diagnostic and therapeutic options. Endoscopy of the small bowel may be ileoscopy as part of colonoscopy, or with enteroscopes which traverse the proximal jejunum (push enteroscopy). The maximum distance of jejunum attainable is in the region of 150 cm. The technique of 'push-pull' or 'double-balloon' enteroscopy makes it possible to visualise the entire small bowel. A long enteroscope and an overtube are used, both of which have an inflatable balloon used to anchor their position in the small bowel.[34] The endoscopist can progress along the small bowel by advancing the enteroscope and the overtube alternately. The small bowel may be approached from either or both ends, with an India-ink tattoo to mark the point reached. If the procedure is performed based on findings of another study, then it may not be necessary to view the entire bowel. Advantages and disadvantages are summarised in Table 6.

Various series have been published showing good results; for instance, finding the source of bleeding in 50 of 66 (76%) obscure GI bleeding patients.[35] Protagonists indiate the procedure is well-tolerated but rare perforations have been reported in abnormal small bowel.[35] It is not commonly available in the UK, but is seen in the US, Germany and Japan. Enteroscopy may be superior to capsule endoscopy in mucosal visualisation,[36] but capsule endoscopy will be effective along the entire length of the small bowel. Future developments may include the concept of virtual enteroscopy to match virtual colonoscopy, although little has been published to date.

Table 6 Advantages and disadvantages of enteroscopy

Advantages
- Therapeutic and biopsy options
- Mucosal visualisation better

Disadvantages
- Invasive
- Risks of bleeding and perforation
- Lower patient acceptability
- Expertise limited

> **Key point 6**
>
> - Push enteroscopy permits therapeutic intervention but has limited reach. Double balloon enteroscopy may overcome this but is very invasive and not widely available.

CAPSULE ENDOSCOPY

Direct luminal visualisation is achieved by the patient swallowing a capsule containing a video camera, microchip and transmitter, with images transmitted to a receiver worn by the patient. The technique is expensive: the single-use capsules cost in the region of £300, the receiver many thousands of pounds, and the image interpretation is time-consuming, taking up to several hours of a gastroenterologist's time. Complications include impaction of the capsule, which may require surgical removal. The world experience suggests an impaction rate of 0.75% after more than 10,000 procedures, and this technique is contra-indicated in patients with stricturing Crohn's disease, those with implanted pacemakers and those with swallowing disorders. Future developments include the development of 'patency capsules', capsules with a lactose body which dissolves after approximately 40 h, which are given in order to confirm patency of the lumen. Retention is checked for by plain abdominal X-ray or a purpose-built portable scanner. Biopsy is not possible at present.[11] With ever greater experience of capsule endoscopy, more small bowel pathology will be visible such as that constituting NSAID-related enteropathy. It remains to be seen what will be the impact of commonly uncovering abnormalities rarely found before. This could result in the diagnosis of previously unrecognised abnormalities leading to further investigations, not all of which may be necessary. Alternatively, new progress may be made in the understanding of disease processes (Fig. 9).

Table 7 Advantages and disadvantages of capsule endoscopy

Advantages
- Direct mucosal visualisation
- Patient acceptability
- Lack of ionising radiation

Disadvantages
- Cost
- Reporting time
- Impaction, possibly requiring surgical removal
- Difficult to localise lesions, as peristaltic speed may vary
- High miss rate

A recent meta-analysis has compared the yield of capsule endoscopy with other imaging modalities in non-stricturing Crohn's disease.[37] Eleven studies involving 309 patients were included.[38–48] In 8 of 11 trials, patients served as their own controls, by undergoing capsule endoscopy within a median of 5 weeks of the comparative study. Seven studies compared capsule endoscopy with small bowel follow-through, two capsule endoscopy with small bowel enema, four capsule endoscopy with colonoscopy and ileoscopy, three with CT enteroclysis, two with enteroscopy and one with MR. Significantly, patients with stricturing disease, seen on a study to assess patency for capsule endoscopy, were excluded from the trials. This suggests that patients included in the studies may have milder disease.

Of the nine studies comparing capsule endoscopy and small bowel contrast studies (SBCS),[38–46] six included patients with suspected Crohn's disease, and

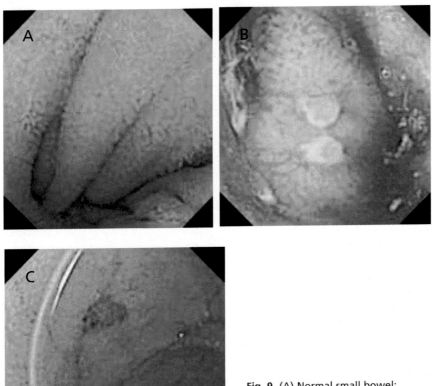

Fig. 9 (A) Normal small bowel; (B) small bowel with Crohn's disease; (C) small bowel with angioectasia.

seven studies included patients being followed up for known Crohn's disease. Overall, when compared with small bowel contrast studies, the yield of capsule endoscopy was 64% versus 24% for findings consistent with Crohn's disease ($P < 0.001$; 95% CI, 28–51%; NNT = 3). For those with suspected Crohn's disease only the yield was 43% for capsule endoscopy and 13% for small bowel contrast studies, which was not statistically significant ($P = 0.09$; 95% CI, –3% to 51%). For those studies concerned with known Crohn's disease, the yield for capsule endoscopy was 78% versus 32% for small bowel contrast studies which was strongly significant ($P < 0.001$; 95% CI, 31–70%; NNT =2).

Three trials compared capsule endoscopy and CT enteroclysis.[38,39,48] Overall yield for capsule endoscopy was 69% compared with 39% for CT enteroclysis ($P = 0.001$; 95% CI, 15–60%). In the suspected Crohn's patients, yield for capsule endoscopy was 70% versus 21%, which became statistically insignificant when the random-effects model was applied ($P = 0.07$; 95% CI, –3% to 80%). For patients with known Crohn's disease, capsule endoscopy yield was 68% versus 38% for CT enteroclysis/enterography ($P = 0.001$; 95% CI, 12–48%). One trial compared capsule endoscopy to MR,[47] but the number was small (two patients with suspected and 16 with known Crohn's disease);

with a diagnostic yield of 72% for capsule endoscopy versus 50% for MR, the difference was not statistically significant ($P = 0.16$; 95% CI, –9% to 53%).

Two trials compared capsule endoscopy with push enteroscopy in suspected and known Crohn's disease.[44,45] Overall yield was 46% versus 8% in favour of capsule endoscopy ($P = 0.001$; 95% CI, 26–50%). However, results were skewed by a relative lack of findings with either test in the suspected Crohn's disease group. This gave non-significant results ($P = 0.51$; 95% CI, –15 to 30%). In the known Crohn's disease group, there was a significant difference ($P < 0.001$; 95% CI, 53–85%). Four trials compared ileocolonoscopy with capsule endoscopy.[39,40,43,44] Overall yield for capsule endoscopy was 61% compared with 46% for colonoscopy with ileoscopy ($P = 0.02$; 95% CI, 2–27%; NNT = 7). In the suspected Crohn's patients, yield for capsule endoscopy was 33% versus 26%, which was not significantly different ($P = 0.48$; 95% CI, –12% to 25%). For patients with known Crohn's disease, capsule endoscopy yield was 86% versus 60% for ileocolonoscopy ($P = 0.002$; 95% CI, 9–43%; NNT = 4).

It is of note that, in patients with suspected Crohn's disease, capsule endoscopy did not give rise to a significantly greater yield over any modality, whereas it did in the known Crohn's disease patients. This is most likely to be due to the heterogeneity of patients labelled as 'suspected Crohn's disease'. It is likely that yields in these studies will be higher than in common clinical practice as these suspected Crohn's disease patients had to fit eligibility criteria to enter their respective trials. Additionally, there is a lack of consensus as to what constitutes Crohn's disease on capsule endoscopy. There is no other gold standard than clinical follow-up, as biopsy is not possible. However, it may be hard to distinguish between Crohn's disease and NSAID-induced enteropathy or other lesions.

No analysis has yet been performed comparing patients with some other objective evidence of Crohn's disease prior to study. The meta-analysis suffers from relatively small numbers in total, but the overall impression is that capsule endoscopy produces a greater yield, and as a 'take-home message' this may be powerful in promoting its uptake in the gastrointestinal world.

Key point 7

- The evidence points towards capsule endoscopy being superior to other imaging modalities in known Crohn's disease. However, it is not used in those with stricturing Crohn's disease patients due to risk of capsule retention. Its usefulness in the patient with suspected Crohn's disease is less clear.

IMPLICATIONS FOR PRACTICE

Radiologists may in the past have found the small bowel unrewarding to image. With a diverse group of patients referred, yields are low. Images may not be discussed with clinical colleagues, in contrast with the multidisciplinary approach to cancer imaging. As with much in medicine, people with dedicated interest are required to develop services. Ideally, a multidisciplinary negotiation should occur at an early stage to decide which tests to develop, followed by regular progress meetings.

From the current literature, a gold standard service would have several tiers of investigation, reflecting the availability, efficacy, expense and expertise required. A department should be encouraged to ultrasound the terminal ileum of patients who present with irritable bowel syndrome-type symptoms, in whom it is desired to exclude inflammatory bowel disease. Ultrasonography should be performed by GI radiologists expert in the field of bowel ultrasonography. The next tier of investigation should be CT enterography or enteroclysis, which should replace barium enteroclysis, as results are similar but the latter is more comprehensive. Rigorous audit should accompany the change in practice, to ensure standards remain high and that results are as good as enteroclysis.

For Crohn's disease patients who may require repeated investigations over many years, MR enteroclysis should be developed. Finally, capsule endoscopy should be available for diagnostic conundrums and the investigation of lesions such as angiodysplasia which are not well seen on cross-sectional imaging. Recommendations for the investigation of obscure GI bleeding have been largely established[49] and are likely to comprise upper and lower GI endoscopy, followed by a repeat UGI endoscopy as lesions are found at enteroscopy that would be within reach of the initial study. This can be followed by capsule endoscopy, then enteroscopy.

Key points for clinical practice

- The small bowel is difficult to image and studies of all techniques are limited by the lack of a gold standard reference and agreed criteria for referral.

- Barium contrast studies are widely available but yield is low.

- Ultrasonography may be very useful and acceptable in identifying terminal ileitis, particularly in children, but its use is very observer-dependent and expertise in bowel ultrasound is not widely available.

- Computed tomography enteroclysis should be at least as good as small bowel enema, and will provide extraluminal information. Images are static and repeated studies, such as Crohn's patients might expect during a life-time, may result in considerable exposure to ionising radiation.

- MR enteroclysis may be equivalent to other imaging modalities, but with the advantage of dynamic imaging and no ionising radiation.

- Push enteroscopy permits therapeutic intervention but has limited reach. Double balloon enteroscopy may overcome this but is very invasive and not widely available.

- The evidence points towards capsule endoscopy being superior to other imaging modalities in known Crohn's disease although it cannot be used in a large subsection of Crohn's disease patients due to stricturing with consequent risk of capsule retention. Its usefulness in suspected Crohn's disease is less clear.

ACKNOWLEDGEMENTS

The authors thank Dr Nick Hennessy, Consultant Radiologist, and Drs Trevor Smith and Sean Weaver, Consultant Gastroenterologists, Royal Bournemouth Hospital, Bournemouth, Dorset, UK.

References

1. Underhill BM. Intestinal length in man. *BMJ* 1955; **2**: 1243–1246.
2. Thomson JN, Hemmingway JP, MacPherson GAD *et al*. Obscure gastrointestinal haemorrhage of small bowel origin. *BMJ* 1984; **288**: 1663–1665.
3. Moch A, Herlinger H, Kochman ML *et al*. Enteroclysis in the evaluation of obscure gastrointestinal bleeding. *AJR Am J Roentgenol* 1994; **163**: 1381–1384.
4. Wills JS, Lobis IF, Denstman FJ. Crohn disease: state of the art. *Radiology* 1997; **202**: 597–610.
5. Maglinte DDT, Chernish SM, Kelvin FM, O'Connor KW, Hage JP. Crohn disease of the small intestine: accuracy and relevance of enteroclysis. *Radiology* 1992; **184**: 541–545.
6. Carlson HC. Perspective: The small bowel examination in the diagnosis of Crohn's disease. *AJR Am J Roentgenol* 1986; **147**: 63–65.
7. Ott DJ, Chen YM, Gelfand DW *et al*. Detailed oral small bowel exam vs. enteroclysis. *Radiology* 1985; **7**: 121–125.
8. Bernstein CN, Boult IF, Greenberg HM *et al*. A prospective randomized comparison between small bowel enteroclysis and small bowel follow-through in Crohn's disease. *Gastroenterology* 1997; **113**: 390–398.
9. Schreyer AG, Golder S, Seitz J *et al*. New diagnostic avenues in inflammatory bowel disease. *Dig Dis* 2003; **21**: 129–137.
10. Dixon PM, Roulston ME, Nolan DJ. The small bowel enema: a ten year review. *Clin Radiol* 1993; **47**: 46–48.
11. MacKalski BA, Bernstein CN. New diagnostic imaging tools for inflammatory bowel disease. *Gut* 2006; **55**: 733–741.
12. Cirillo LC, Camera L, Della Noce M *et al*. Accuracy of enteroclysis in Crohn's disease of the small bowel: a retrospective study. *Eur Radiol* 2000; **10**: 1894–1898.
13. Bremner AR, Griffiths M, Argent JD, Fairhurst JJ, Beattie RM. Sonographic evaluation of inflammatory bowel disease: a prospective blinded comparative study. *Pediatr Radiol* 2006; **36**: 947–953
14. Bremner AR, Pridgeon J, Fairhurst J, Beattie RM. Ultrasound scanning may reduce the need for barium scanning in the assessment of small-bowel Crohn's disease. *Acta Paediatr* 2004; **93**: 479–481.
15. Fraquelli M, Colli A, Casazza G *et al* Role of US in detection of Crohn disease: meta-analysis. *Radiology* 2005; **236**: 95–101.
16. Calabrese E, La Seta F, Buccellato A *et al*. Crohn's disease: a comparative prospective study of transabdominal ultrasonography, small intestine contrast ultrasonography and small bowel enema. *Inflamm Bowel Dis* 2005; **11**: 139–145.
17. Parente F, Greco S, Molteni M *et al*. Oral contrast enhanced bowel ultrasonography in the assessment of small intestine Crohn's disease. A prospective comparison with conventional ultrasound, X-ray studies and ileocolonoscopy. *Gut* 2004; **53**: 1652–1657.
18. Yekeler E, Danalioglu A, Movaseghi B *et al*. Crohn disease activity evaluated by Doppler ultrasound of the superior mesenteric artery and the affected small bowel segments. *J Ultrasound Med* 2005; **24**: 59–65.
19. Byrne MF, Farrell MA, Abass S *et al*. Assessment of Crohn's disease by Doppler ultrasonography of the superior mesenteric artery, clinical evaluation and the Crohn's disease clinical activity index: a prospective study. *Clin Radiol* 2001; **56**: 973–978.
20. Hassan C, Cerro P, Zullo A *et al*. Computed tomography enteroclysis in comparison with ileoscopy in patients with Crohn's disease. *Int J Colorect Dis* 2003; **18**: 121–125.
21. Boudiaf M, Jaff A, Soyer P *et al*. Small bowel diseases: prospective evaluation of multi-detector row helical CT enteroclysis in 107 consecutive patients. *Radiology* 2004; **233**: 338–344.
22. Orjollet-Lecoanet C, Ménard Y, Martins A *et al*. CT enteroclysis for detection of small

bowel tumours. *J Radiol* 2001; **81**: 618–627.

23. Minordi LM, Vecchioli A, Guidi L *et al*. Multidetector CT enteroclysis versus barium enteroclysis with methylcellulose in patients with suspected small bowel disease. *Eur Radiol* 2006; **16**: 1527–1536.

24. Sailer J, Peloschek R, Schober E *et al*. Diagnostic value of CT enteroclysis compared with conventional enteroclysis in patients with Crohn's disease. *AJR Am J Roentgenol* 2005; **185**: 1575–1581.

25. Paulsen SR, Huprich JE, Fletcher JG *et al*. CT enterography as a diagnostic tool in evaluating small bowel disorders: review of clinical experience with over 700 cases. *Radiographics* 2006; **26**: 641–662.

26. Mazzeo S, Caramella D, Battolla L *et al*. Crohn disease of the small bowel: spiral CT evaluation after oral hyperhydration with isotonic solution. *J Comput Assist Tomogr* 2001; **25**: 612–616.

27. Masseli G, Brizi GM, Parella B *et al*. Crohn disease: magnetic resonance enteroclysis. *Abdom Imaging* 2004; **29**: 329–334.

28. Maglinte DDT, Siegleman ES, Kelvin FM. MR enteroclysis: the future of small bowel imaging? *Radiology* 2000; **215**: 639–641.

29. Masselli G, Brizi MHG, Menchini L *et al*. Magnetic resonance enteroclysis imaging of Crohn's. *Radiol Med (Torino)* 2005; **110**: 221–233.

30. Low RN, Francis IR, Pollitoske D, Bennett M. Crohn's disease evaluation: comparison of contrast-enhanced MR imaging and single phase helical CT scanning. *J Magn Reson Imaging* 2000; **11**: 127–135.

31. Wiarda BM, Kuipers EJ, Houddijk LP *et al*. MR enteroclysis: imaging technique of choice in diagnosis of small bowel diseases. *Dig Dis Sci* 2004; **50**: 1036–1040.

32. Masselli G, Casciani E, Polettini E *et al*. Assessment of Crohn's disease in the small bowel: prospective comparison of magnetic resonance enteroclysis with conventional enteroclysis. *Eur Radiol* 2006; **16**: 2817–2827.

33. Gourtsoyiannis NC, Grammatikakis J, Papamastorakis G *et al*. Imaging of small intestinal Crohn's disease: comparison between MR enteroclysis and conventional enteroclysis. *Eur Radiol* 2006; **16**: 1915–1925.

34. Gerson LB. Double-balloon enteroscopy: the new gold standard for small bowel imaging? *Gastrointest Endosc* 2005; **62**: 71–75.

35. Yamamoto H, Kita H, Sunada K *et al*. Clinical outcomes of double-balloon endoscopy for diagnosis and treatment of small-intestinal diseases. *Clin Gastroenterol Hepatol* 2004; **2**: 1010–1016.

36. Appleyard M, Fireman Z, Glukhovsky A *et al*. A randomized trial comparing wireless capsule endoscopy with push enteroscopy for the detection of small bowel lesions. *Gastroenterology* 2000; **119**: 1431–1438.

37. Triester SL, Leighton JA, Leontiadis GI *et al*. A meta-analysis of the yield of capsule endoscopy compared to other diagnostic modalities in patients with non-stricturing small bowel Crohn's disease. *Am J Gastroenterol* 2006; **101**: 954–964.

38. Eliakim R, Suissa A, Yassin K *et al*. Wireless capsule video endoscopy compared to barium follow-through and computerised tomography in patients with suspected Crohn's disease – Final report. *Dig Liver Dis* 2004; **36**: 519–522.

39. Hara AK, Leighton JA, Heigh RI *et al*. Crohn's disease of the small bowel: preliminary comparison of CT enterography, capsule endoscopy, small-bowel follow-through and ileoscopy. *Radiology* 2006; **238**: 128–134.

40. Bloom P, Rosenberg M, Klein S *et al*. Wireless capsule endoscopy is more informative than ileoscopy and SBFT for the evaluation of the small intestine in patients with known or suspected Crohn's disease [Abstract]. Second International Conference on Capsule Endoscopy – Changing Clinical Practice, March 2003, Berlin, Germany.

41. Buchman AL, Miller FH, Wallin A *et al*. Video capsule endoscopy versus barium contrast studies for the diagnosis of Crohn's disease recurrence involving the small intestine. *Am J Gastroenterol* 2004; **99**: 2171–2177.

42. Costamagna G, Shah SK, Riccioni ME *et al*. A prospective trial comparing small bowel radiographs and video capsule endoscopy for suspected small bowel disease. *Gastroenterology* 2002; **123**: 999–1005.

43. Dubcenco E, Jeejeebhoy KN, Petroniene R *et al*. Diagnosing Crohn's disease of the small

bowel: should capsule endoscopy be used? CE vs. other diagnostic modalities. *Gastrointest Endosc* 2004; **59 (Suppl S)**: AB 174.

44. Toth E, Fork FT, Almqvist P *et al*. Wireless capsule enteroscopy: a comparison with enterography, push enteroscopy and ileo-colonoscopy in the diagnosis of small bowel Crohn's disease. *Gastrointest Endosc* 2004; **59 (Suppl S)**: AB 173.

45. Chong AKH, Taylor A, Miller A *et al*. Capsule endoscopy vs. push enteroscopy and enteroclysis in suspected small-bowel Crohn's disease. *Gastrointest Endosc* 2005; **61**: 255–261.

46. Marmo R, Rotondano G, Bianco MA *et al*. Wireless capsule endoscopy vs. small bowel enteroclysis in the detection of ileal involvement in Crohn's disease: a prospective controlled trial. *Gastrointest Endosc* 2004; **59 (Suppl S)**: AB 177.

47. Golder SK, Schreyer AG, Endlicher E *et al*. Comparison of capsule endoscopy and magnetic resonance (MR) enteroclysis in suspected small bowel disease. *Int J Colorect Dis* 2006; **21**: 97–104.

48. Voderholzer WA, Beinhoelzl J, Rogalla P *et al*. Small bowel involvement in Crohn's disease: a prospective comparison of wireless capsule endoscopy and computed tomography enteroclysis. *Gut* 2005; **54**: 369–373.

49. Sidhu R, Sanders DS, McAlindon ME. Gastrointestinal capsule endoscopy: from tertiary centres to primary care. *BMJ* 2006; **332**: 528–531.

Tahseen Qureshi Daniel O'Leary Amjad Parvaiz

10

Laparoscopic surgery for colorectal cancer: current practice and training

In 1901, George Kelling performed the first experimental laparoscopy by insufflating air into the peritoneum of a dog, visualising the cavity with a cystoscope.[1] Although the first publications on laparoscopy appeared from a French surgeon, Raoul Palmer, the leading pioneer of laparoscopic surgery was Professor Kurt Semm.[2] Despite initial ridicule, he persisted with his innovative ideas on minimally invasive surgery from the 1960s and went on to perform the first laparoscopic appendicectomy in the 1980s.[3] The first laparoscopic cholecystectomy was performed by Muhe in 1985[4] but limits in instrumentation meant the first laparoscopic colonic resections were not performed until 5 years later, a laparoscopic right hemicolectomy by Jacobs.[5] Later that year, Fowler performed the first laparoscopic sigmoid resection[6] and this was followed soon after by the first resection of a rectal cancer by Leahy.[7]

Although laparoscopic cholecystectomy was rapidly adopted by the surgical community, the evolution of laparoscopic colorectal surgery has been slow, accounting for less than 10% of colorectal resections in most countries.[8] The explanation is partly due to resistance from surgeons themselves. As with so many technical developments, laparoscopic colorectal surgery was initially greeted with a muted response. It was variously viewed as a 'triumph of technology over common sense', oncologically unsound, too time consuming, too expensive or too difficult to learn. With time, persistence, evidence, and effort, the position has changed dramatically. Most colorectal units now want

Tahseen Qureshi FRCS FRCS(Gen Surg)
Fellow Laparoscopic Colorectal Surgery, Queen Alexandra Hospital, Portsmouth, PO6 3LY, UK

Daniel O'Leary BSc FRCS FRCS(Gen)
Consultant Colorectal Surgeon, Queen Alexandra Hospital, Portsmouth, PO6 3LY, UK

Amjad Parvaiz FRCS FRCS(Gen Surg) (for correspondence)
Consultant Colorectal Surgeon, Centre for Training in Laparoscopic Colorectal Surgery, Queen Alexandra Hospital, Southwick Hill Road, Cosham, Portsmouth, PO6 3LY, UK
E-mail: amjad.parvaiz@porthosp.nhs.uk

to develop and provide laparoscopic colorectal surgery and more and more colorectal surgeons want to do it. The remaining issue is how to train them.

CURRENT STATUS

It is useful to analyse the factors that have brought about this change in attitude. They include: (i) technical advances; (ii) evidence of oncological safety; (iii) belief that it is good for patients; and (iv) patient demand.

TECHNICAL ADVANCES

Surgeons in many countries have now developed the necessary laparoscopic skills and operative strategies to complete complex colorectal operations to a standard that is as good as, or better, than can be achieved by conventional operating techniques. Much of this results from the determination of a few pioneers who have pushed the boundaries while maintaining safety. Developments in imaging with a three chip camera system and high-definition technology have been crucial. Design of atraumatic bowel graspers and stapling devices for minimally invasive surgery have made possible more technically demanding operations. Better dissecting and haemostatic technology, including LigasureTMTM, Harmonic Scalpel and conventional diathermy mean that it is now possible to dissect tissue planes more easily as haemostasis is almost absolute. These technical developments have made it easier for surgeons to carry out laparoscopic colorectal operations and this, in turn, has made it easier and more reasonable to generalise the techniques within the surgical community.

> ## Key point 1
>
> - Technical advances mean that laparoscopic colorectal surgery can be performed under ideal operating conditions.

EVIDENCE OF ONCOLOGICAL SAFETY

Early reports of metastases at port sites and extraction sites stifled enthusiasm for laparoscopic resections for colorectal cancer.[9] In the UK, they were one factor which led the National Institute for Health and Clinical Excellence (NICE) to advise that laparoscopic colectomy for cancer should only be undertaken in the context of appropriately designed clinical trials. Intense scrutiny by the surgical community backed up by laboratory research led to improved operative techniques for handling the bowel and use of wound protectors to protect the extraction site from contamination by tumour. As a result, recent publications have reported an incidence of wound or port-site metastasis similar to that in open surgery.[10–12] This should no longer be an issue.

Subsequent investigations have shown that laparoscopic resections for colorectal cancer produce adequate lymph node yields and tumour clearance, without any detrimental effect on complications, mortality, local recurrence or long-term survival.[13–18]

The degree to which operations are completed laparoscopically is variable and may be difficult to ascertain in individual publications. Laparoscopically-assisted and hand-assisted operations are not the same as an entirely laparoscopic operation with intracorporeal vascular ligation, mobilisation of colon and intra- or extracorporeal anastomosis. We regard the procedure to be a conversion if an incision is made to facilitate dissection rather than for specimen extraction or extracorporeal anastomosis.

A number of randomised controlled trails and studies have looked into the safety and feasibility of laparoscopic colorectal surgery.

MRC CLASICC trial[19]

This trial of Conventional vs Laparoscopic Assisted Surgery In Colorectal Cancer randomised 794 patients in the UK with either colon or rectal cancer; 268 and 526 were randomised to open and laparoscopic surgery, respectively. There were no differences between the groups in terms of rate of positive resection margins (CRMs), proportion of Dukes' C2 tumours, in-hospital mortality, intra-operative and postoperative complications and quality of life over 3 months. Complications were higher for rectal resections (13% versus 7%) and those who underwent a conversion ($P = 0.002$). A non-significant increase in positive CRM was seen for lap anterior resection for rectal cancer compared to open surgery (12% versus 6%; $P = 0.19$). However, surgeons early in their learning curve qualified for inclusion (minimum of 20 resections).

COST trial[12]

This American multicentre trial (Clinical Outcomes of Surgical Therapy Study Group) included 48 centres and 872 patients with colonic cancer randomised to either laparoscopically assisted or open surgery. With a median follow up of 4.4 years, there was no significant difference in the rate of tumour recurrence (16% laparoscopic versus 18% open; $P = 0.32$). The overall survival rate at 3 years was also similar between the two groups (86% laparoscopic versus 85% open; $P = 0.51$). Conversion rates were high at 21%, indicative of surgeons at the beginning of their laparoscopic experience.

COLOR trial[20]

The COlon Carcinoma Laparoscopic or Open Resection trial was a randomised European multicentre study with 1248 patients in each group. The primary end-point was cancer-free survival 3 years after surgery. Patients assigned laparoscopic resection had less blood loss compared with those assigned open resection (median 100 ml versus 175 ml; $P < 0.0001$), although laparoscopic surgery lasted 30 min longer than open surgery ($P < 0.0001$). Conversion to open surgery was needed for 91 (17%) patients undergoing the laparoscopic procedure. Adequacy of resection, assessed by lymph node yield and length of resection margins, did not differ between the groups. The laparoscopic group had an earlier recovery of bowel function ($P < 0.0001$), needed less analgesia and required a shorter hospital stay ($P < 0.0001$) when compared with the open group. Morbidity and mortality 28 days after colectomy did not differ between groups. They concluded that laparoscopic surgery was safe for cancer in the right, left, and sigmoid colon

Other trials and meta-analyses

Lacey et al.[11] published perhaps the most interesting results. They randomised 219 patients with colonic cancer to either laparoscopically assisted or open surgery. With a median follow-up of 43 months, the rate of tumour recurrence, site of recurrence and overall survival were not significantly different between the two groups. However, the cancer-related survival was significantly higher in the laparoscopic group and stratification according to tumour stage showed that this difference was due to improved outcomes in stage III disease. In patients with stage III disease, the laparoscopic group had significantly better results for tumour recurrence, overall survival and cancer related survival.

Morino et al.[21] published a prospective study examining 100 consecutive patients treated with laparoscopic total mesorectal excision (TME). After a median follow-up of nearly 4 years, there was a single port site metastasis and the overall locoregional recurrence rate was 4.2%. This compares well with open TME.

Abraham et al.[67] reported a meta-analysis of short-term outcomes after laparoscopic resection for colorectal cancer. Twelve randomised controlled trials (RCTs) were considered, a total of 2512 patients. They concluded the following: (i) adequate cancer clearance in both groups; (ii) laparoscopic procedures took longer (> 30%); (iii) laparoscopic morbidity rate was at least 30% lower; (iv) haemorrhage/blood transfusion, re-operation, cardiorespiratory complications and anastomotic leaks favoured the laparoscopic group (did not reach statistical significance); (v) quicker gastrointestinal and respiratory recovery in laparoscopic surgery; (vi) laparoscopic surgery associated with less pain, requiring less narcotic analgesia; and (vii) shorter hospital stay after laparoscopic surgery.

Key points 2 & 3

- Good evidence indicates that laparoscopic surgery for carcinoma of the colon and rectum can be done safely, with good early outcomes.

- Cancer-related outcomes are at least as good as with conventional surgery 3–4 years after operation.

LAPAROSCOPIC COLORECTAL SURGERY IS GOOD FOR PATIENTS

Patients undergoing laparoscopic resection for colorectal cancer in many institutions can have the same oncological operation performed as with conventional surgery. The benefits are indicated in Table 1. A Cochrane review (2005) concluded that laparoscopic colonic resections conferred benefit with respect to both medical and surgical morbidity.

Although the operating costs are greater in laparoscopic surgery, a recent systematic review showed that total hospital costs are similar; indeed, there may be lower indirect costs for laparoscopic colorectal surgery. They concluded that cost should not be a deterrent to performing laparoscopic colorectal surgery.[22]

Table 1 Advantages of laparoscopic colorectal resection for cancer versus conventional operation[11,18,53–61]

Advantage	Reference(s)
Small incisions	62,63
Reduced blood loss	11,54,57
Reduced pain	18,57
Better pulmonary function after operation	57
Earlier return of gut function	64
Earlier mobilisation	11,18,55
Earlier discharge	18,65
Fewer complications	66
Enhanced quality of life at 30 days	53

Laboratory correlates

Laboratory studies support the clinical impression that laparoscopic operations are less traumatic to the patient. This is reflected in reduced production of interleukins 6 and 10, indicating a reduced physiological stress response. However, the clinical significance of a reduction in the immune response remains unclear.[23] Patients with colorectal cancer have elevated levels of serum vascular endothelial growth factor, a potent angiogenesis factor.[24] Levels rise after open surgery, but the increase is less after laparoscopic surgery.[25]

Laparoscopic colorectal resection and enhanced recovery programmes

The ethos of enhanced recovery is 'maintenance of normality' in the peri-operative period, thereby modifying the stress response.[26,27] Enhanced recovery programmes are multimodal and applicable to open and laparoscopic colorectal surgery. Pre-operatively, patients are given carbohydrate-rich drinks, to avoid postoperative insulin resistance, and they are taught stoma care if defunctioning is anticipated. The use of epidurals and avoidance of opiates as pain killers allows early return of gut function and fewer problems with postoperative nausea and vomiting. All tubes, drains and catheters are removed by the second postoperative day. The results seen by the originators in Denmark have been reproduced by others, including a group practising laparoscopic colorectal surgery with an enhanced recovery program in the UK.[28]

Key point 4

- Laparoscopic surgery can contribute to the development of an enhanced recovery surgical programme.

PATIENT DEMAND AND EXPECTATIONS

Working in a hospital that is making the change from open to laparoscopic colorectal surgery, it is apparent that patients want the minimally invasive operation. The attention of the mass media, patient support groups, information on the Internet and patients themselves has focused attention on 'keyhole' surgery. Patients want minimally invasive surgery because of the perceived advantages, notably faster recovery and smaller scars. However, it is also clear that they expect high quality and expect to be treated by fully trained surgeons who are competent in what they are offering.

SUMMARY OF CURRENT PRACTICE

It is now accepted that laparoscopic resection for colorectal cancer can achieve equivalent oncological results to conventional surgery. In addition, there may be significant advantages as indicated above. Current NICE guidance (2006) supports laparoscopic colorectal resection by appropriately trained and experienced surgeons.[29]

The UK Department of Health has indicated that it wants all hospitals that carry out colorectal surgery for bowel cancer to offer laparoscopic resections by 2009 and to achieve laparoscopic resections in 50% of their patients by 2012. The key question now is not if colorectal surgery should be done laparoscopically, but whether and how it can be generalised to the community of colorectal surgeons currently in practice. The objective is no less than retraining a generation of colorectal surgeons in a new way of operating for the benefit of their patients.

IMPLEMENTATION OF TRAINING

NICE has recommended that laparoscopic colorectal resections for malignancy be performed only by surgeons who have completed the appropriate training.[29] Recognised pathways for training in laparoscopic colorectal surgery are evolving. Currently, trainees may apply for ALSGBI/ACPGBI sponsored fellowships in four different units in the UK. Each fellowship lasts 6 months and trainees are expected to undertake colonic resections independently by the end of their training. In addition, some centres offer training fellowships sponsored by industry. It is expected that as more consultants develop skills in laparoscopic colorectal surgery their trainees would have undertaken the straightforward colonic resections during their rotation and the fellowships in specialist units would evolve to provide training in more complex laparoscopic colorectal surgery including rectal cancer surgery.

For existing consultants, the ALS/ACPGBI offers a Preceptorship Programme in which consultants are trained and supervised through laparoscopic colorectal operations by approved, experienced colorectal laparoscopic surgeons so that their initial experiences in this field are safe and effective. The UK Department of Health has just launched a pilot project to set up 10 Minimally Invasive Surgery Training Centres for Colorectal Cancer with the aim of training existing consultant colorectal surgeons in techniques for laparoscopic colorectal cancer resection.

This national programme gives a powerful impetus to the development of laparoscopic colorectal surgery in the UK.

Key point 5

- Training programmes are available for the safe introduction of laparoscopic colorectal surgery.

Key to its success will be an understanding of laparoscopic learning, appropriate selection of candidates for training, a structured training methodology, clearly defined end points of training, assessment of competence and structures or processes for further training and maintenance of competence. Validation and revalidation will feature. These issues will be considered in turn.

LAPAROSCOPIC LEARNING

The term 'learning curve' originates from aircraft manufacture.[30] It came to prominence in the 1980s following the introduction of laparoscopic cholecystectomy. Laparoscopic cholecystectomy spread quickly, without quality assurance, resulting in an increase in bile duct injuries and criticism from the academic community due to the lack of controlled prospective studies. However, the precise definition of a learning curve in surgery is not clear. Parameters such as 'time to independence', 'operating time', 'complication rate', 'hospital stay' and 'mortality' have all been used to characterise the process.[31] More recently, multidimensional assessment of learning curves has been recommended.[32] However defined or measured, the effect of the learning curve is cumulative, allowing performance to be plotted as a curve. Practice improves performance generating a 'steep' phase to the learning curve before performance plateaus at a level which will differ between individuals.[33]

Factors affecting the learning curve

The type of training received and characteristics of the individual surgeon influence the shape of the learning curve and final competence. Training on inanimate simulators as well as animal tissue facilitates learning.[34] A surgeon's skill acquisition is not related to the surgeon's age, size of practice or hospital setting.[35] However, some authors have observed that the complication rate reciprocates the surgical workload.[36] Surgeons need to perform 25–30 cases before becoming proficient at laparoscopic fundoplication[37–40] in contrast to a threshold of about 15–20 cases for laparoscopic cholecystectomy.[41–44] It seems likely that skills obtained in one minimal access procedure do not necessarily transfer to others.

It follows that surgeons who can carry out laparoscopic cholecystectomy do not qualify to perform laparoscopic colonic resections without first undergoing additional training specifically in laparoscopic colorectal techniques.[45,46]

IMPLICATIONS FOR COLORECTAL SURGERY

For many procedures, the surgeon's learning curve has been characterised;[47–49] however, in laparoscopic colorectal surgery, the number of cases required before a surgeon reaches the plateau is not clear.[32] It is recognised that this surgery is difficult to perform and requires advanced laparoscopic skills and considerable experience. Schlachta et al.[50] have suggested that fellowship training provides enough experience such that the issues surrounding a surgeon's learning curve are redundant when he or she starts their own practice. In their series, the conversion rate of a fellowship-trained surgeon was no higher than that of a more experienced surgeon. Surgeons who perform higher volumes of laparoscopic colectomies have lower rates of intra- and postoperative complications.[51] Laparoscopic operations for colon cancer at hospitals with high caseloads appear to be associated with improved short-term results.[52]

Key point 6

- The provision of fellowships in high-volume colorectal centres facilitates rapid learning of laparoscopic surgical techniques.

SELECTION OF TRAINEES

Competence in open colorectal surgery and possession of core generic laparoscopic skills shortens the learning curve for colorectal resections. There is a step-wise progression of required laparoscopic skills before performing more complex procedures. Diagnostic laparoscopy, laparoscopic appendicectomy, laparoscopic cholecystectomy, laparoscopic stoma formation and laparoscopic inguinal/incisional hernia repair all offer invaluable experience in the acquisition of the laparoscopic skills that are fundamental to advanced laparoscopic colorectal operations.

STRUCTURED TRAINING METHODOLOGY

A preceptored model of training is favoured. Initially, this requires trainees to observe and assist several laparoscopic colorectal resections. This is supported by the development or refinement of core competencies and knowledge in a surgical skills or laparoscopic skills laboratory.

Hands-on preceptored training then follows, with the trainee surgeon performing laparoscopic surgery under the direct supervision of a preceptor surgeon who assists at the operation.

Most colorectal procedures lend themselves to a modular approach to teaching. For example a colorectal resection can be divided into a number of stages.

1. Patient set-up and creation of a pneumoperitoneum.
2. Vascular pedicle isolation and control.
3. Colonic mobilisation.
4. Exteriorisation and anastomosis (extra- or intracorporeal).
5. Closure.

Careful case selection is important for training. The ideal patient for a training operation will have a body mass index (BMI) < 28 kg/m^2, no previous abdominal surgery, no major co-morbidity, and a high sigmoid or caecal neoplasm. High anterior resection and right hemicolectomy are the easier laparoscopic resections to learn and to teach. Laparoscopic resection for lesions of the transverse colon, splenic flexure, distal sigmoid or rectum is technically demanding and should be avoided during the initial phase of learning or independent practice.

COMPETENCE ASSESSMENT

After the supervised training period, the challenge is to determine whether the trainee is ready for independent practice. To date, no such core curriculum or accreditation process is in place to sign off the trainees. Development of an appropriate competence assessment is important: methods of assessment and standards to reach should be agreed nationally. It is likely that parameters to assess would include:

- appropriateness of case selection
- ability to complete the steps of a laparoscopic colorectal resection in a safe, stepwise, logical manner as observed by one or more non-scrubbed preceptors/assessors
- manual dexterity and selection of instruments
- identification of dissection planes and anatomy
- recognition of intra-operative difficulty
- understanding of strategies to deal with intra-operative difficulty
- insight into ability and limitations
- willingness to seek advice/convert to open operation
- patient safety
- relationships with the theatre team.

At least for a time, the range of complexity of laparoscopic colorectal operations will mean that many surgeons will focus on completing the easier right and left colectomies laparoscopically and will continue to perform conventional operations for low rectal cancer and other complex pelvic conditions. Surgeons with better developed laparoscopic skills will develop a practice in these more difficult areas, perhaps in larger centres.

Conversion to open surgery should not be regarded as a failure, but instead should demonstrate good judgement on the part of the surgeon. The key in making the decision is the timing of conversion. Published evidence has shown that patients who had late conversion tended to have worse outcomes when compared with those who either have the procedure completed laparoscopically or an early conversion. Different surgeons will develop at a different pace and the number of procedures required to be competent will be variable. The current preceptor programme in the UK requires 20 cases to be completed by the surgeon under training before he or she can be signed off to perform laparoscopic surgery independently.

With appointment of national centres for training in laparoscopic colorectal surgery, it is expected that a core curriculum and assessment tools would be in place to enable trainees to be signed off for their competence.

Key point 7

- Competence assessment must be part of any training programme, but requires standards to be agreed.

TRAINING THE TEAM

Laparoscopic colorectal surgery is very much a team effort. It requires that all who are involved in the care of the patient take an active part. This includes pre-operative counselling so that the patient knows what to expect and, in particular, how to facilitate their own recovery. The anaesthetist and theatre team need to be trained to understand the demands of positioning for laparoscopic colorectal surgery, positioning of stacks and monitors, the availability of appropriate instruments and advanced haemostatic dissecting tools. Finally, this surgery requires a commitment to train theatre personnel and to maintain the equipment in working order. Postoperatively, the patient should be nursed on a ward that runs an enhanced recovery programme, with a judicious selection of analgesic regimens, avoiding opiates. A number of centres now run 'Laparoscopic Colorectal Masterclasses'. This provides the opportunity for the whole operating team to visit a unit where such practice is routine.

CONCLUSIONS

Laparoscopic colorectal surgery is now well established. Initial concerns about its oncological safety and costs have been resolved. Oncologically sound, laparoscopic colorectal resection is likely to become the gold standard for colorectal cancer. Training is now the key issue if the experience of specialist units is to be generalised for the benefit of patients everywhere. Training opportunities are improving. The challenge is to provide structured training in laparoscopic colorectal surgery to trainees and existing colorectal surgeons so that they may progress their learning curve in a preceptored manner without detriment to patients. Ultimately, the majority of elective colorectal surgery may be completed laparoscopically. We envisage that with careful, safe, preceptored training, this standard can be achieved throughout the UK.

Key points for clinical practice

- Technical advances mean that laparoscopic colorectal surgery can be performed under ideal operating conditions.
- Good evidence indicates that laparoscopic surgery for carcinoma of the colon and rectum can be done safely, with good early outcomes.
- Cancer-related outcomes are at least as good as with conventional surgery 3–4 years after operation.
- Laparoscopic surgery can contribute to the development of an enhanced recovery surgical programme.
- Training programmes are available for the safe introduction of laparoscopic colorectal surgery.
- The provision of fellowships in high-volume colorectal centres facilitates rapid learning of laparoscopic surgical techniques.
- Competence assessment must be part of any training programme, but requires standards to be agreed.

References

1. Gunning JE, Rosenzweig BA. Evolution of endoscopic surgery. In: White RA, Klein SR. (eds) *Endoscopic Surgery*. Boston, MA: Mosby Year Book, 1991; p1–9.
2. Litynski GS. Kurt Semm and an automatic insufflator. *J Soc Laparoendosc Surg* 1998; **(2)**: 197–200.
3. Tuffs A. Obituary Kurt Semm. *BMJ* 2003; **327**: 397.
4. Jani K, Rajan PS, Sendhilkumar K, Palanivelu C. Twenty years after Erich Muhe: persisting controversies with the gold standard of laparoscopic cholecystectomy. *J Min Access Surg* 2006; **2**: 49–58.
5. Jacobs M, Verdeja JC, Goldstein HS. Minimally invasive colon resection. *Surg Laparosc Endosc* 1991; **1**: 144–150.
6. Fowler DL, White SA, Anderson CA. Laparoscopic colectomy – 60 cases. *Surg Laparosc Endosc* 1995; **5**: 468–471.
7. Sgambati SA, Ballantyne GH. History of minimally invasive colorectal surgery. In: Rama M, Jager RM, Wexner SD. (eds) *Laparoscopic Colorectal Surgery*. New York: Churchill Livingstone, 1995, pp13–23.
8. Motson RW. Laparoscopic surgery for colorectal cancer. *Br J Surg* 2005; **92**: 519–520.
9. Berends FJ, Kazemier G, Bonjer HJ, Lange JF. Subcutaneous metastases after laparoscopic colectomy. *Lancet* 1994; **58**: 344.
10. Vukasin P, Ortega AE, Greene FL *et al*. Wound recurrence following lap colon cancer resection. Results of the American Society of Colon and Rectal Surgeons Laparoscopic Registry. *Dis Colon Rectum* 1996; **39 (Suppl 10)**: S20–S23.
11. Lacy AM, Garcia-Valdecasas JC, Delgado S *et al*. Laparoscopy-assisted colectomy versus open colectomy for treatment of non-metastatic colon cancer; a randomised control trial. *Lancet* 2002; **359**: 2224–2229.
12. Clinical Outcomes of Surgical Therapy Study Group. A comparison of laparoscopically assisted and open colectomy for colon cancer. *N Engl J Med* 2004; **350**: 2050–2059.
13. Tate JJ, Kwok S, Dawson JW, Lau WY, Li AK. Prospective comparison of laparoscopic and conventional anterior resection. *Br J Surg* 1993; **80**: 1396–1398.
14. Ota DM, Nelson H, Weeks JC. Controversies regarding laparoscopic colectomy for malignant diseases. *Curr Opin Gen Surg* 1994; 732–740.
15. Lacy AM, Garcia-Valdecasas JC, Pique JM *et al*. Short term outcome analysis of a randomised study comparing laparoscopic versus open colectomy for colon cancer. *Surg Endosc* 1995; **9**: 1101–1105.
16. Fine AP, Lanasa S, Gannon MP, Cline CW, James R. Laparoscopic colon surgery: report of a series. *Ann Surg* 1995; **61**: 412–416.
17. Lord SA, Larach SW, Ferrara A, Williamson PR, Lago CP, Lube MW. Laparoscopic resections for colorectal carcinoma. A three year experience. *Dis Colon Rectum* 1996; **39**: 148–154.
18. Stage JG, Schulze S, Moller P *et al*. Prospective randomised study of laparoscopic versus open colonic resection for adenocarcinoma. *Br J Surg* 1997; **84**: 391–396.
19. Guillou PJ, Quirke P, Thorpe H *et al*. CLASICC trial. *Lancet* 2005; **365**: 1718–1726.
20. Veldkamp R, Kuhry E, Hop WC *et al*. Laparoscopic surgery versus open surgery for colon cancer: short-term outcomes of a randomised trial. *Lancet Oncol* 2005; **6**: 477–484.
21. Morino M, Parini U, Giraudo G *et al*. Laparoscopic total mesorectal excision: a consecutive series of 100 patients. *Ann Surg* 2003; **237**: 335–342.
22. Dowson HM, Huang A, Soon Y, Gage H, Lovell DP, Rockall TA. Systematic review of the costs of laparoscopic colorectal surgery. *Dis Colon Rectum* 2007; **50**: 908–919.
23. Ng CSH, Whelan RL, Lacy AM, Yim AP. Is minimal access surgery for cancer associated with immunological benefits? *World J Surg* 2005; **29**: 975–981.
24. Yoo J, Laparoscopic colorectal surgery. *Permanente J* 2008; **12**: 27–31.
25. Belizon A, Balik E, Feingold DL *et al*. Major abdominal surgery increases plasma levels of vascular endothelial growth factor: open more so than minimally invasive methods. *Ann Surg* 2006; **244**: 792–798.
26. Kehlet H. Multimodal approach to control postoperative pathophysiology and rehabilitation. *Br J Anaesth* 1997; **78**: 606–617.
27. Kehlet H, Wilmore DW. Multimodal strategies to improve surgical outcome. *Am J Surg* 2002; **183**: 630–641.

28. King PM, Blazeby JM, Ewings P, Kennedy RH. A randomised control trial comparing laparoscopic and open surgery for colorectal cancer within an enhanced recovery programme. *Br J Surg* 2006; **93**: 300–308.

29. National Institute for Health and Clinical Excellence. Guidance on the use of laparoscopic surgery for colorectal cancer. Technology Appraisal Guidance No 105. London: NICE, 2006.

30. Subramonian K, Muir G. The learning curve in surgery: what is it, how do we measure it and can we influence it? *BJU Int* 2004; **93**: 1173–1174.

31. Michel LA. Epistelogy of evidence-based medicine. *Surg Endosc* 2007; **21**: 146.

32. Dincler S, Koller MT, Steurer J, Bachman LM, Christen D, Buchmann P. Multi-dimensional analysis of learning curves in laparoscopic sigmoid resection: eight year results. *Dis Colon Rectum* 2003; **46**: 1371–1378.

33. Cook JA, Ramsay CR, Fayers P. Statistical evaluation of learning curve effect in surgical trials. *Clin Trials* 2004; **1**: 421–427.

34. Traxer O, Gettman MT, Wapper CA *et al.* The impact of intense laparoscopic skills training on the operation performance of urology residents. *J Urol* 2003; **166**: 1658–1661.

35. Gibbs VC, Auerbach AD. Learning curve for new procedures – the case of Laparoscopic Cholecystectomy Health Services/Technology Assessment Text. Chapter 19 (online) http//:www.ahrq.gov/clinic/ptsafety/chap19.

36. Hu J, Gold KF, Pashos CL, Mehtas, Litwin MS. Role of surgeon volume in radical prostatectomy outcomes. *J Clin Oncol* 2003; **21**: 401–405.

37. Champault GG, Barrat C, Rozon RC, Rizk N, Catheline JM. The effect of the learning curve on the outcome of laparoscopic treatment for gastroesophageal reflux. *Surg Laparosc Endosc Percutan Tech* 1999; **9**: 375–381.

38. Watson DI, Baigrie RJ, Jamieson GG. A learning curve for laparoscopic fundoplication. Definable, avoidable, or a waste of time? *Ann Surg* 1996; **224**: 198–203.

39. Soot SJ, Eshraghi N, Farahmand M, Sheppard BC, Deveney CW. Transition from open to laparoscopic fundoplication: the learning curve. *Arch Surg* 1999; **134**: 278–281.

40. Deschamps C, Allen MS, Trastek VF, Johnson JO, Pairolero PC. Early experience and learning curve associated with laparoscopic Nissen fundoplication. *J Thorac Cardiovasc Surg* 1998; **115**: 281–288.

41. Zucker KA, Bailey RW, Gadacz TR, Imbembo AL. Laparoscopic guided cholecystectomy. *Am J Surg* 1991; **161**: 36–42.

42. A prospective analysis of 1518 laparoscopic cholecystectomies. The Southern Surgeons Club. *N Engl J Med* 1991; **324**: 1073–1078.

43. Moore MJ, Bennett CL. The learning curve for laparoscopic cholecystectomy. The Southern Surgeons Club. *Am J Surg* 1995; **170**: 55–59.

44. Gigot J, Etienne J, Aerts R *et al.* The dramatic reality of biliary tract injury during laparoscopic cholecystectomy. An anonymous multicentre Belgian survey of 65 patients. *Surg Endosc* 1997; **11**: 1171–1178.

45. Grundfest WS. Credentialing in an era of change. *JAMA* 1993; **270**: 2725.

46. Agachan F, Joo JS, Weiss EG, Wexner SD. Intraoperative laparoscopic complications. Are we getting better? *Dis Colon Rectum* 1996; **39**: S14–S19.

47. Agachan F, Joo JS, Sher M, Weiss EG, Nogueras JJ, Wexner SD. Laparoscopic colorectal surgery. Do we get faster? *Surg Endosc* 1997; **11**: 331–335.

48. Schlachta CM, Mamazza J, Seshadri PA, Cadeddu M, Gregoire R, Poulin EC. Defining the learning curve for laparoscopic colorectal resection. *Dis Colon Rectum* 2001; **44**: 217–222.

49. Perino A, Cucinella G, Venezia R, Castelli A, Cittadini E. Total laparoscopic hysterectomy versus total abdominal hysterectomy: an assessment of the learning curve in a prospective randomised study. *Hum Report* 1999; **14**: 2996–2999.

50. Schlachta CM, Mamazza J, Gregoire R, Burpe SE, Pace KT, Poulin EC. Predicting conversion in laparoscopic colorectal surgery. Fellowship training may be an advantage. *Surg Endosc* 2003; **17**: 1288–1291.

51. Bennett CL, Stryker SJ, Ferreira MR, Adams J, Beart RW. The learning curve for laparoscopic colorectal surgery. Preliminary results from a prospective analysis of 1194 laparoscopic-assisted colectomies. *Arch Surg* 1997; **132**: 41–44.

52. Kuhry E, Bonjer HJ, Haglind E *et al.* Impact of hospital case volume on short-term outcome after laparoscopic operation for colonic cancer. *Surg Endosc* 2005; **19**: 687–692.

53. Schwenk W, Haase O, Neudecker J, Müller JM. Short term benefits for laparoscopic colorectal resection. Cochrane Database of Syst Rev 2005; Issue 3. Art. No.: CD003145.

54. Kiran RP, Delaney CP, Senagore AJ, Millward BL, Fazio VW. Operative blood loss and use of blood products after laparoscopic and conventional open colorectal operations. *Arch Surg* 2004; **139**: 39–42.

55. Leung KL, Kwok SPY, Lam SCW *et al*. Laparoscopic resection of rectosigmoid carcinoma: prospective randomised trial. *Lancet* 2004; **363**: 1187–1192.

56. Delaney CP, Kiran RP, Senagore AJ, Brady K, Fazio VW. Case-matched comparison of clinical and financial outcome after laparoscopic or open colorectal surgery. *Ann Surg* 2003; **238**: 67–72.

57. Milsom JW, Bohm B, Hammerhofer KA, Fazio V, Steiger E, Elson P. A prospective randomised trial comparing laparoscopic versus conventional techniques in colorectal cancer surgery: a preliminary report. *J Am Coll Surg* 1998; **187**: 46–54.

58. Braga M, Vignali A, Gianotti L *et al*. Laparoscopic versus open colorectal surgery: a randomised trial on short-term outcome. *Ann Surg* 2002; **236**: 759–766.

59. Duepree HJ, Senagore AJ, Delaney CP, Fazio VW. Does means of access affect the incidence of small bowel obstruction and ventral hernia after bowel resection? Laparoscopy versus laparotomy. *J Am Coll Surg* 2003; **197**: 177–181.

60. Psaila J, Bulley SH, Ewings P, Sheffield JP, Kennedy RH. Outcome following laparoscopic resection for colorectal cancer. *Br J Surg* 1998; **85**: 662–664.

61. Weeks JC, Nelson H, Gelber S, Sargent D, Schroeder G. Short-term quality-of-life outcomes following laparoscopic-assisted colectomy versus open colectomy for colon cancer (for the COST study group). *JAMA* 2002; **287**: 321–328.

62. Ramos JM, Beart Jr RW, Goes R *et al*. Role of laparoscopy in colorectal surgery. A prospective evaluation of 200 cases. *Dis Colon Rectum* 1995; **38**: 494–501.

63. Dunker MS, Stiggelbout AM, van Hogezand RA *et al*. Cosmesis and body image after laparoscopic assisted and open ileocolic resection for Crohn's disease. *Surg Endosc* 1998; **12**: 1334–1340.

64. Chen HH, Wexner SD, Iroatulam AJ *et al*. Laparoscopic colectomy compares favourably with colectomy by laparotomy for reduction of post-operative ileus. *Dis Colon Rectum* 2000; **43**: 61–65.

65. Lacy AM, Garcia-Valdecasas JC, Pique JM *et al*. Short-term outcome analysis of a randomised study comparing laparoscopic versus open colectomy for colon cancer. *Surg Endosc* 1995; **9**: 1101–1105.

66. Dwivedi A, Chahin F, Agrawal S *et al*. Laparoscopic colectomy versus open colectomy for sigmoid diverticular disease. *Dis Colon Rectum* 2002; **45**: 1309–1314.

67. Abraham NS, Young JM, Solomon MJ. Meta-analysis of short-term outcomes after laparoscopic resection for colorectal cancer. *Br J Surg* 2004; **91**: 1653–1654.

Rowan J. Collinson   Neil J. McC. Mortensen

11

TEMS for tumours of the rectum

It is almost a quarter of a century since transanal endoscopic microsurgery (TEMS) was first reported by Buess and colleagues from Cologne for the management of tumours of the mid-to-lower rectum.[1] From its initial status as a promising but expensive and technically-demanding procedure, it now has an established role in the management of benign tumours. It has an expanding role in the management of malignant tumours also, a role which demands an expert understanding of the nature of local recurrence, metastasis and the place of adjuvant therapies.

Tumours of the mid-to-lower rectum have always proved problematic for the surgeon. A compromise must always be achieved between minimising morbidity and mortality, while achieving adequate clearance of the lesion, especially if it is malignant. It is not surprising, therefore, that a range of procedures is described in the literature, from Parks' transanal excision,[2] to locally morbid operations such as the trans-sphincteric and trans-sacral approaches of Mason and Kraske, respectively,[3] through finally to transabdominal proctectomy, with or without permanent stoma. TEMS allows the surgeon to work in anatomical planes, with excellent vision, while exploiting the less morbid transanal approach.

EQUIPMENT

TEMS utilises a 4-cm diameter operating proctoscope which comes in 12-cm and 20-cm lengths and incorporates a bevelled end. The face plate of the TEMS

Rowan J. Collinson FRACS (for correspondence)
Clinical Colorectal Research Fellow, Department of Colorectal Surgery, GI Physiology Unit, Level 2, The John Radcliffe Hospital, Headley Way, Headington, Oxford OX3 9DU, UK
E-mail: rowan.collinson@ntlworld.com

Neil J. McC. Mortensen MD FRCS
Professor of Colorectal Surgery, The John Radcliffe Hospital, Headley Way, Headington, Oxford OX3 9DU, UK

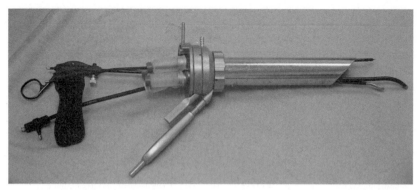

Fig. 1 Assembled TEMS proctoscope.

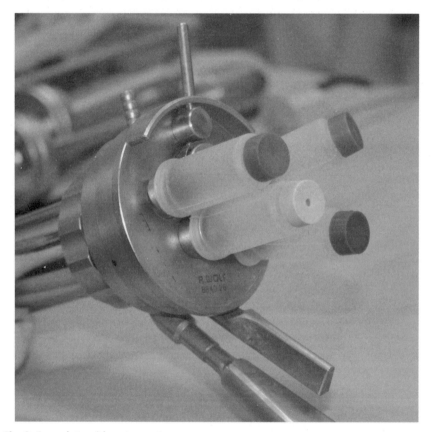

Fig. 2 Face plate with entry ports.

proctoscope seals to provide not only a closed system allowing carbon dioxide insufflation, but also four entry ports for a range of instruments (Figs 1 and 2). These include a suction/irrigation unit, graspers, a needle point diathermy, and needle holders for suturing. Once inserted, the operating proctoscope is held in fixed position by the Martin arm clamp. The operator can utilise a binocular optical system with x6 magnification, or a camera which feeds to television screens within the operating room.

TECHNIQUE

Full bowel preparation and intravenous antibiotics are given pre-operatively. The procedure is performed under general anaesthesia, preferably with muscle relaxation to avoid respiratory movement. The tumour must always be orientated inferiorly. Therefore, for anterior tumours, the patient is placed in prone jack-knife position with legs apart; for posterior tumours, the lithotomy position is used. Following assembly and insertion of the TEMS proctoscope, a margin of at least 5 mm around the tumour is scored with diathermy. A submucosal or full-thickness resection of the tumour can then be performed. If there is any possibility of malignancy, full-thickness resection is required, although progress into the mesorectal fat is minimised, to avoid compromising any subsequent transabdominal total mesorectal excision if this is found to be necessary after histological review. The tumour is removed and pinned out on a cork board for orientation. The residual rectal wound can be left open, or closed with a running suture secured with metal clips at each end.

INDICATIONS

The ideal lesion for TEMS is an adenoma within 20 cm of the anal verge. More specifically, the lesion must be below the peritoneal reflection, to avoid entry into the peritoneal cavity in a full-thickness excision. Therefore, 12 cm is the approximate limit anteriorly (Fig. 3). Adenomas of this description are typically large, flat lesions not amenable to colonoscopic polypectomy, and may even be circumferential. While there is no definite size restriction, larger adenomas should be removed by full-thickness excision, due to the risk of harbouring a malignancy.

TEMS is also indicated for selected rectal cancers. This decision is based on the likelihood of lymph node metastases, since tumours with potential lymph

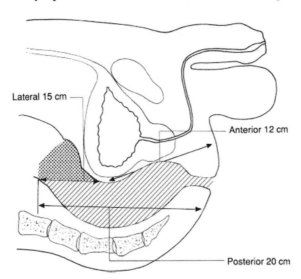

Lateral 15 cm

Anterior 12 cm

Posterior 20 cm

Fig. 3 The 'safe' area for resection of rectal lesions. Hatched area, all tumours; stippled area, care should be taken anteriorly and laterally beyond 12 cm. Reproduced, with permission, from Cook and Mortensen.[34]

Table 1 T1 tumours and risk factors for lymph node metastases

	'Low risk'	'High risk'
Degree of differentiation	Well/moderate	Poor
Histological grade	1 and 2	3
Histological subtype		Mucinous adenocarcinoma
Lymphovascular space invasion	–	+
Kikuchi et al.[5] level	sm1	sm2 and sm3
Tumour diameter	< 3 cm	≥ 3 cm

node involvement must undergo a conventional cancer operation (*i.e.* low anterior resection [LAR] or abdominoperineal resection [APR]) including lymphadenectomy. The suitability of a cancer for TEMS is assessed on radiological and histological criteria.

Endorectal ultrasound (ERUS) is the preferred imaging modality, as the T-stage of the cancer is crucial. ERUS is particularly suited to the important distinction between T1 and T2 tumours, with an accuracy of 82–93% in the published literature.[25] Magnetic resonance imaging (MRI) is poor at this discrimination and, in the lower rectum, MRI has difficulty even making the distinction between T2 and T3 tumours. MRI can provide valuable information about the status of mesorectal lymph nodes. The accuracy of MRI in detecting lymph node metastasis ranges from 72–92%, compared to 65-81% for ERUS.[31] Therefore, in practical terms, ERUS and MRI are complementary in assessing the suitability of a rectal cancer for TEMS excision.

Histological criteria are based on the work of Hermanek and Gall,[4] and the depth of invasion as defined by Kikuchi et al.[5] The work of both relates to early colorectal cancer, defined as tumour whose invasion is limited to submucosa (T1). Early rectal cancers at high risk for lymph node metastases are histological grade 3 adenocarcinomas or mucinous adenocarcinomas, or undifferentiated tumours, and those with lymphovascular space invasion. Kikuchi et al.[5] divided T1 tumours into sm1, sm2 and sm3, depending on the depth of submucosal invasion. sm1 tumours are defined as those with < 300 μm of invasion into submucosa. The authors did not demonstrate lymph node involvement in sm1 tumours. Therefore, the ideal cancers for TEMS as the definitive procedure are small, well-differentiated adenocarcinomas with no lymphovascular space invasion and minimal invasion of the submucosa (Table 1).

Key points 1 & 2

- Radiological work-up of rectal malignancies must include both endorectal ultrasound and magnetic resonance imaging of the tumour and mesorectum if local excision is contemplated.

- Reproducible histological criteria can divide early rectal cancers into low risk and high risk of lymph node involvement, and this is essential to the planning of therapy.

MORBIDITY AND MORTALITY

An obvious benefit of TEMS is decreased operative morbidity and mortality, when compared with conventional surgery. This appears self-evident in the case of cancer, when the other options (LAR or APR) clearly have more complications (Table 2), and are associated with an approximate 5% mortality rate.[40] By contrast, the morbidity rate of TEMS is approximately 4%,[13] with the most common being fever, bleeding, suture line dehiscence, intraperitoneal perforation and urinary retention. However, even in the case of benign lesions of the low rectum where the alternative operation would be a standard transanal resection, TEMS also has benefits, such as a decreased rate of local recurrence,[13] most likely due to the increased operative precision.

It is clear that there is little clinically-relevant impact upon sphincter function, despite the prolonged anal sphincter dilatation with the 4-cm operating proctoscope. A significant decrease in anal resting pressure at 6–12 weeks' postoperatively has been demonstrated,[6–8] but this does not seem to translate into significant impairment of continence scores or quality of life.[6,9] Distinct internal sphincter damage visible on endosonography has been reported by some,[8,10] but discounted by others.[6] Pre-operative incontinence and long operative time (> 2 h) have been implicated as risk factors for postoperative incontinence,[6,10] highlighting the need for adequate pre-operative assessment, particularly in the elderly. However it is suggested that any iatrogenic sphincter impairment may have recovered by 6 months' postoperatively.[8]

Table 2 Incidence of morbidity following anterior resection

• Urinary dysfunction	7–68%
• Sexual impotence	15–100%
• Absent ejaculation	3–39%
• Dyspareunia	18–90%
• Anastomotic leak	5–10%
• Mortality	4–6%

From Nastro et al.[40]

COST EFFECTIVENESS

The favourable morbidity profile of TEMS makes the procedure highly cost-effective.[11,12] In the large experience reported by Maslekar and Monson,[12] the cost per TEMS case (for benign and malignant disease) was compared with that of matched controls undergoing conventional open abdominal surgery (LAR/APR). The cost per patient for a TEMS case was £567, compared with

Key point 3

- Transanal endoscopic microsurgery (TEMS) has an excellent morbidity and mortality profile when compared with conventional abdominal surgical approaches to low rectal tumours.

£4135 per open operation. The authors point out that this easily justifies the initial expenditure for the TEMS equipment (at approximately £40,000).

Key points 4 & 5

- There is no evidence of clinically significant impairment of anal continence following TEMS surgery.
- Despite high set-up costs, TEMS is a highly cost-effective approach to low rectal tumours.

ADENOMAS

TEMS is now an established modality for dealing with adenomas of the rectum. The reach of the equipment up to 20–25 cm from the anal verge is superior to that of other transanal approaches.[2] The precise excision afforded may explain the low rates of local recurrence. A review by Maslekar et al.[13] reported a mean local recurrence rate of 4.5% (range, 0–11%) across 18 case series, with 1857 patients. Similar figures have been reported in several recent large series not included in that analysis.[14–17] In the only randomised trial of TEMS versus peranal submucosal excision for adenoma, Winde et al.[18] reported a local recurrence rate of 6% and 22%, respectively. Of note, this study also compared TEMS and anterior resection for T1 cancer[35] (see below).

Size of the lesion and completeness of excision are the key determinants of local recurrence.[16,17] In particular, McCloud et al.[16] found that their early recurrences (within 6 months) were all in incompletely excised cases, as were the majority of their late recurrences. They concluded that a follow-up programme can, therefore, be modified by the excision results, with early endoscopy only for incompletely excised cases.

Giant adenomas (> 5 cm diameter) can be successfully removed with TEMS.[19,20] As stated above, there is a greater risk of local recurrence. Ideally they should incorporate a full-thickness excision due to the increased risk of harbouring a malignancy,[13] although caution must be excised in the upper rectum where entry into the peritoneal cavity is possible.

Key point 6

- TEMS is a safe and established modality for dealing with mid-to-low rectal adenomata, especially those beyond the reach of traditional transanal excision.

CARCINOMAS

T1 TUMOURS

It remains unclear whether any T-stage of invasive cancer can or should be treated definitively with TEMS. At the forefront of this debate is the T1 lesion.

In practice, excision of a T1 lesion with TEMS typically occurs in one of two ways. A patient may undergo TEMS for a presumed adenoma, and a focus of early invasive cancer is subsequently identified in the specimen on definitive histology. Alternatively, pre-operative biopsy may suggest malignancy in a clinically and radiologically early lesion. In this circumstance, the TEMS procedure can serve as a large biopsy to obtain definitive evidence of invasion. In both of these circumstances, if the lesion is well-differentiated, with clear margins and no evidence of lymphovascular space invasion (*i.e.* a 'low-risk' lesion), a dilemma arises as to whether any further treatment is necessary, or even justifiable, given the potential morbidity of radical surgery. The difficulty lies in quantifying the likelihood of lymph node involvement and the potential for local recurrence.

Hermanek and Gall[4] estimated the rate of lymph node involvement to be 3% in early colorectal cancer, although they commented that this is much lower than the published historical rate at that time (of approximately 12%). Other authors have shown this figure to be anywhere from 0–21% even for the low-risk rectal lesion.[25,31,32] This supports the view that the distal rectum in particular may have a higher propensity to lymph node metastasis for a given T-stage than colon.[32] More recently, Borschitz et al.[21] published a rate of 3% for low-risk and 20% for high-risk T1 lesions. This included a 5% rate of distant metastasis, seen in both low- and high-risk groups. Clearly, this also serves to demonstrate that, even with rigorous tumour and lymph node staging, other hitherto unidentified subtleties of 'bad' tumour biology may also play a role.

The next consideration is local recurrence. Pooled data published in 2006, involving 22 case series with a total of 552 patients showed a mean local recurrence rate of 6% (range, 0–13%) for T1 lesions excised with TEMS.[13] Stratification for low- and high-risk lesions was not possible. The median follow-up was 21 months (range, 7–41 months). Data from more recent case series concur with this, with local recurrence of 7.5–10% reported from three further centres.[15,22,23] Borschitz et al.[21] stratified their 105 T1 lesions into low and high risk, and found a 6% and 20% local recurrence rate, respectively, with a median follow-up of 74 months. Data from the Swedish Rectal Cancer Registry were also published in 2007: 643 local excisions of rectal cancer over a 6-year period were reported.[24] Stage I lesions had a cumulative 5-year local recurrence rate of 7.2%, although the proportions of T1 and T2 lesions were not stated.

Therefore, the data seem to indicate that for the low-risk T1 cancer the local recurrence rate is at the most approximately 6%. Enthusiasts for the local excision of T1 cancers use this argument to support their practice. However, it must always be kept in mind that the gold standard for the patient treated with curative intent still remains the Dutch rectal cancer trial data, which demonstrated a 0.7% local recurrence rate at 2 years for T1–T2 tumours treated with LAR alone.[33]

One randomised prospective study has compared TEMS with anterior resection for T1 tumours.[35] Poorly differentiated tumours were excluded. The anterior resection group contained 28 patients with a mean 45.8 months' follow-up, while the TEMS group contained 25 patients with 40.9 months' follow-up. There was no difference in local recurrence between anterior resection and TEMS (0 of 28 and 1 of 25), and no difference in mortality (1 of

28 and 1 of 25). However, it is likely that this study is underpowered, and, therefore, must be interpreted with caution.

> ## Key point 7
>
> - Local recurrence and lymph node metastasis rates for T1 tumours are significant, even with low-risk rectal tumours, and the gold standard for cure remains total mesorectal excision.

Salvage surgery

One option for managing local recurrence after local excision is planned salvage surgery. This usually takes the form of a conventional LAR or APR. 'Salvage' can occur in two situations – either as immediate re-operation (usually in the case of a confirmed high-risk T1 excised at TEMS), or delayed re-operation when local recurrence actually occurs (usually in the situation of an originally 'low-risk' tumour). In the latter situation, the local recurrence is usually confined to the rectal wall.[25] Immediate re-operation decreases the chance of local recurrence when compared to TEMS then observation,[31] but has not been shown to affect disease-free survival. Despite this, immediate re-operation carries a greater likelihood of 5-year disease-free survival than delayed re-operation,[31,36] and is, therefore, the preferred option.

Borschitz et al.[21] have recently published their series of 105 patients with pT1 carcinomas (Table 3). They offered immediate radical re-operation to their 'Group B' patients – those with high-risk histology, R1 resection, tumour fragmentation at removal, or tumour ≤ 1 mm from the resection margin. 'Group A' patients (low-risk histology and R0 resection) were observed and re-operated only with confirmed recurrence during an intensive follow-up period. Median follow-up was 74 months. Not all patients in Group B underwent re-operation, and 4 patients in Group A elected for radical surgery rather than observation. The best 5-year cancer-free survival figures were found in 'Group A TEMS only' and 'Group B TEMS and re-operation', with 94% and 93%, respectively. The local recurrence rate in each of these situations was 6%. The worst 5-year cancer-free survival figures were predictably seen in the 'Group B TEMS only' patients (57%), with a local recurrence rate of > 20%.

Table 3 Cancer-free survival (CFS) after TEMS alone and after TEMS with re-operation

Histology	Procedure	Patients (n)	Mean age (years)	CPS (%) 5 yrs	CPS (% 10 yrs	α
Group A	TEMS	66	66 (41–81)	94	89	P = 0.162
	TEMS and re-operation	4	60 (47–67)	75	75	
Group B	TEMS	18	68 (49–86)	57	49	P = 0.015
	TEMS and re-operation	17	60 (39–81)	93	93	

From Borschitz et al.[21]
Cancer-free survival CFS

The 'Group A radical re-operation' patients had intermediate 5-year cancer-free survival. This paper makes two important points. First, should an unexpected high-risk T1 be found after TEMS, it would appear that immediate salvage surgery can reduce the risk of local recurrence to that of TEMS for a low-risk lesion, and similarly affect 5-year cancer-free survival. Second, a local recurrence rate of 6% for a low-risk T1 cancer is arguably still too high.

Therefore, current opinion remains divided on the optimal surgical management of T1 lesions. Concerns have been raised about the possible undertreatment of these patients.[39] Postoperative adjuvant radiotherapy may present a useful adjunct, although it remains relatively unexplored. This may be due to the validation of neo-adjuvant treatment in the setting of total mesorectal excision, although this is arguably not an equivalent situation. However, adjuvant radiotherapy with or without chemotherapy has been shown to decrease the local recurrence rate and increase time to local recurrence for locally excised T1 tumours.[37,38] In one study, this was found to be independent of histological high-risk factors.[38]

Key point 8

- Optimal TEMS technique does not compromise subsequent salvage surgery, and this is most advantageous when performed as an immediate re-operation.

T2–T3 TUMOURS

There is more consensus in the management of T2–T3 lesions. The local recurrence rate for TEMS alone for T2 lesions was estimated to be 14% by Maslekar et al.,[13] although they noted that the data are derived from small series and variable follow-up. When all local excision techniques are considered, the local recurrence rate for T2 is even higher, at approximately 25%.[25] Moreover, the rate of lymph node metastases is 16–40%.[4] For T3 lesions resected by TEMS, a local recurrence rate of approximately 20% has been observed.[13] Therefore, it is clear that TEMS alone is inappropriate for patients with T2–T3 tumours being treated with curative intent. However, TEMS may still play a role in the palliative management of patients with symptomatic T2 and T3 lesions, or in combination with neo-adjuvant therapy for patients treated with curative intent.

Neo-adjuvant treatment

There is a growing interest in neo-adjuvant radiotherapy or combination chemoradiotherapy in the setting of TEMS. Patients have been treated at all T-stages, although this treatment approach seems most relevant to T2 and early T3 lesions. An absolute requirement is the absence of lymph node involvement on pre-operative radiological staging if the patient is being treated with curative intent with TEMS. Response to the neo-adjuvant treatment appears to be an important indicator of the likelihood of local recurrence following TEMS.

Previous studies on rectal cancer have shown a complete pathological response rate of up to 30%.[26] These patients have an excellent prognosis, even in the absence of surgical treatment.[27]

Lezoche et al.[28] recently published their experience with combined modality treatment. A total of 100 patients with T2 and T3 tumours of the extraperitoneal rectum underwent standard neo-adjuvant radiotherapy or chemoradiotherapy followed by TEMS. Tumour diameter was specified at < 3 cm. Pre-operative imaging included endorectal ultrasound, and MRI or CT scan to exclude regional and distant disease. The TEMS excision was full-thickness including mesorectal fat, down to mesorectal fascia, to produce a 'truncated pyramid'-shaped specimen. The authors noted no difficulty closing the rectal wall defect despite the radiotherapy, and noted 8 suture line dehiscences in subsequent follow-up. Median follow-up was 55 months. The cumulative probability of local recurrence and distant recurrence at 90 months' follow-up (Kaplan–Meier method) was 5% and 2%, respectively. The authors noted that no recurrence occurred in any patient whose tumour was down-staged, or down-sized by > 50% following neo-adjuvant treatment. They stated that this was the most reliable prognostic indicator of success.[28] Another study only offered TEMS to patients who showed a 'significant' response to neo-adjuvant therapy, based on clinical and radiological criteria.[29] They reported one local recurrence (who subsequently underwent APR) in their 8 patients and no lymph node or distant metastases following TEMS, during a median 37 months' follow-up. Patients with tumours of any T-stage were allowed to enter this trial, although numbers were too small to draw any statistically significant conclusions.

Lezoche et al.[30] have also published the only randomised prospective trial of T2 tumours undergoing laparoscopic total mesorectal excision or TEM after standard neo-adjuvant therapy. There were 35 patients in each arm, with a minimum of 5 years' follow-up (median, 84 months). Unsurprisingly, operative time, length of stay, intra-operative blood loss and need for transfusion were significantly greater in the laparoscopic group, although overall morbidity was the same. The local recurrence rate for laparoscopic and TEM patients was the same at 6% and 9%, respectively. Again, the local and systemic failures were seen only in patients who did not have a significant response to radiotherapy. Disease-free survival was 94% for both groups at the end of 5 years' minimum follow-up. While this would seem to support the transanal approach, it must be kept in mind that, once again, the local recurrence rate in both groups is high, when compared to other trials of neo-adjuvant therapy and optimal radical surgery.

Key points 9 & 10

- TEMS excision alone is inadequate for curative treatment of T2 and T3 malignancies.

- Neo-adjuvant techniques show some promise in this group, but rely on accurate pre-operative staging of local and distant disease.

FUTURE DIRECTIONS

While the technique of TEMS is well-established, further developments can be expected in the indications and applications of neo-adjuvant and adjuvant therapies. Clearly, the ability to predict lymph node involvement in a non- or minimally-invasive way would be a major advantage to the TEMS surgeon. Imaging techniques will continue to improve, but at this stage they are only a surrogate for definitive tissue assessment.

In 2006, Zerz et al.[41] reported the intriguing technique of endoscopic posterior mesorectal excision (EPMR), a minimally invasive technique whereby the posterolateral mesorectum can be excised via a perineal approach to the retrorectal space. EPMR was performed in a series of 11 patients who underwent transanal local excision for low rectal cancer. A median of 8 (range, 4–20) lymph nodes were found in the mesorectal specimen. Two patients (one low-risk T1, one high-risk T1) had a positive node in the specimen. Survival data are reported to a median follow-up of 48 months, with no local recurrence but one death due to hepatic metastases in a male patient with a high-risk tumour and negative nodes in the EPMR specimen. While numbers are too small to draw any conclusions at this stage, it is a technique which shows some promise, particularly for the T1 tumour, which may occupy an uncomfortable middle ground between undertreatment and overtreatment.

CONCLUSIONS

Nearly a quarter of a century on, TEMS is now an established and acceptable modality for dealing with benign tumours of the mid-to-lower rectum. It offers a low morbidity approach that is cost effective and surgically precise. TEMS also has a growing role for malignant tumours of the rectum. Accurate histological analysis is central to this approach. The risk of lymph node metastasis dictates whether TEMS excision alone is adequate or whether salvage surgery or adjuvant therapy is required. Neo-adjuvant techniques show promise, but rely on accurate pre-operative radiological staging. It is important, however, that standards achieved with this minimally invasive approach are benchmarked against the recent progress made in the more radical approaches such as total mesorectal excision.

Key points for clinical practice

- Radiological work-up of rectal malignancies must include both endorectal ultrasound and magnetic resonance imaging of the tumour and mesorectum if local excision is contemplated.

- Reproducible histological criteria can divide early rectal cancers into low risk and high risk of lymph node involvement, and this is essential to the planning of therapy.

- Transanal endoscopic microsurgery (TEMS) has an excellent morbidity and mortality profile when compared with conventional abdominal surgical approaches to low rectal tumours.

(continued)

Key points for clinical practice *(continued)*

- There is no evidence of clinically significant impairment of anal continence following TEMS surgery.

- Despite high set-up costs, TEMS is a highly cost-effective approach to low rectal tumours.

- TEMS is a safe and established modality for dealing with mid-to-low rectal adenomata, especially those beyond the reach of traditional transanal excision.

- Local recurrence and lymph node metastasis rates for T1 tumours are significant, even with low-risk rectal tumours, and the gold standard for cure remains total mesorectal excision.

- Optimal TEMS technique does not compromise subsequent salvage surgery, and this is most advantageous when performed as an immediate re-operation.

- TEMS excision alone is inadequate for curative treatment of T2 and T3 malignancies.

- Neo-adjuvant techniques show some promise in this group, but rely on accurate pre-operative staging of local and distant disease.

References

1. Buess G, Theis R, Gunther M, Hutterer F, Pichlmaier H. Endoscopic surgery of the rectum. *Endoscopy* 1985; **17**: 31–35.
2. Parks AG, Stuart AE. The management of villous tumours of the large bowel. *Br J Surg* 1973; **60**: 688–695.
3. Buess G, Kipfmuller K, Hack D, Grussner R, Heintz A, Junginger T. Technique of transanal endoscopic microsurgery. *Surg Endosc* 1988; **2**: 71–75.
4. Hermanek P, Gall FP. Early (microinvasive) colorectal carcinoma. Pathology, diagnosis, surgical treatment. *Int J Colorect Dis* 1986; **1**: 79–84.
5. Kikuchi R, Takano M, Takagi K *et al*. Management of early invasive colorectal cancer. Risk of recurrence and clinical guidelines. *Dis Colon Rectum* 1995; **38**: 1286–1295.
6. Kennedy ML, Lubowski DZ, King DW. Transanal endoscopic microsurgery excision. Is anorectal function compromised? *Dis Colon Rectum* 2002; **45**: 601–604.
7. Kreis ME, Jehle EC, Haug V *et al*. Functional results after transanal endoscopic microsurgery. *Dis Colon Rectum* 1996; **39**: 1116–1121.
8. Gracia Solanas JA, Ramirez Rodriguez JM, Aguilella Diago V, Elia Guedea M, Martinez Diez M. A prospective study about functional and anatomic consequences of transanal endoscopic microsurgery. *Rev Esp Enferm Dig* 2006; **98**: 234–240.
9. Cataldo PA, O'Brien S, Olser T. Transanal endoscopic microsurgery: a prospective evaluation of functional results. *Dis Colon Rectum* 2005; **48**: 1366–1371.
10. Herman RM, Richter P, Walega P, Popiela T. Anorectal sphincter function and rectal barostat study in patients following transanal endoscopic microsurgery. *Int J Colorectal Dis* 2001; **16**: 370–376.
11. Farmer KC, Wale R, Winnett J, Cunningham I, Grossberg P, Polglase A. Transanal endoscopic microsurgery: the first 50 cases. *Aust NZ J Surg* 2002; **72**: 854–856.
12. Maslekar S, Pillinger SH, Sharma A, Taylor A, Monson JRT. Cost analysis of transanal endoscopic microsurgery for rectal tumours. *Colorect Dis* 2007; **9**: 229–234.
13. Maslekar S, Beral DL, White TJ, Pillinger SH, Monson JRT. Transanal endoscopic microsurgery: where are we now? *Dig Surg* 2006; **23**: 12–22.

14. Guerrieri M, Baldarelli M, Morino M *et al.* Transanal endoscopic microsurgery in rectal adenomas: experience from six Italian centres. *Dig Liver Dis* 2006; **38**: 202–207.

15. Bretagnol F, Merrie A, George B, Warren BF, Mortensen NJ. Local excision of rectal tumours by transanal endoscopic microsurgery. *Br J Surg* 2007; **94**: 627–633.

16. McCloud JM, Waymont N, Pahwa N *et al.* Factors predicting early recurrence after transanal endoscopic microsurgery excision for rectal adenoma. *Colorect Dis* 2006; **8**: 581–585.

17. Whitehouse PA, Tilney HS, Armitage JN, Simson JNL. Transanal endoscopic microsurgery: risk factors for local recurrence of benign rectal adenomas. *Colorect Dis* 2006; **8**: 795–799.

18. Winde G, Schmid KW, Reers B, Bunte H. Microsurgery in prospective comparison with conventional transanal excision or anterior rectum resection in adenomas and superficial carcinomas [in German]. *Langenbecks Arch Chir Suppl Kongressbd* 1996; **113**: 265–268.

19. Said S, Stippel D. Transanal endoscopic microsurgery in large, sessile adenomas of the rectum. A 10-year experience. *Surg Endosc* 1995; **9**: 1106–1112.

20. Schafer H, Baldus SE, Holscher AH. Giant adenomas of the rectum: complete resection by transanal endoscopic microsurgery (TEM). *Int J Colorect Dis* 2006; **21**: 533–537.

21. Borschitz T, Heintz A, Junginger T. The influence of histopathologic criteria on the long-term prognosis of locally excised pT1 rectal carcinomas: results of local excision (transanal endoscopic microsurgery) and immediate reoperation. *Dis Colon Rectum* 2006; **49**: 1492–1506.

22. Floyd ND, Saclarides TJ. Transanal endoscopic microsurgical resection of pT1 rectal tumours. *Dis Colon Rectum* 2005; **49**: 164–168.

23. Stipa F, Burza A, Lucandri G *et al.* Outcomes for early rectal cancer managed with transanal endoscopic microsurgery. A 5-year follow-up study. *Surg Endosc* 2006; **20**: 541–545.

24. Folkesson J, Johansson R, Pahlman L, Gunnarsson U. Population-based study of local surgery for rectal cancer. *Br J Surg* 2007; **94**: 1421–1426.

25. Sengupta S, Tjandra JJ. Local excision of rectal cancer. What is the evidence? *Dis Colon Rectum* 2001; **44**: 1345–1361.

26. Habr-Gama A, de Souza PM, Ribeiro Jr U *et al.* Low rectal cancer: impact of radiation and chemotherapy on surgical treatment. *Dis Colon Rectum* 1998; **41**: 1087–1096.

27. Habr-Gama A, Perez RO, Nadalin W *et al.* Operative versus nonoperative treatment for stage 0 distal rectal cancer following chemoradiation therapy: long-term results. *Ann Surg* 2004; **240**: 711–717.

28. Lezoche E, Guerrieri M, Paganini AM, Baldarelli M, De Santis A, Lezoche G. Long-term results in patients with T2-3 N0 distal rectal cancer undergoing radiotherapy before transanal endoscopic microsurgery. *Br J Surg* 2005; **92**: 1546–1552.

29. Caricato M, Borzomati D, Ausania F *et al.* Complementary use of local excision and transanal endoscopic microsurgery for rectal cancer after neoadjuvant chemoradiation. *Surg Endosc* 2006; **20**: 1203–1207.

30. Lezoche G, Baldarelli M, Paganini AM, De Sanctis A, Bartolacci S, Lezoche E. A prospective randomised study with a 5-year minimum follow-up evaluation of transanal endoscopic microsurgery versus laparoscopic total mesorectal excision after neoadjuvant therapy. *Surg Endosc* 2007; Epub ahead of print.

31. Hahnloser D, Wolff BG, Larson DW, Ping J, Nivatvongs S. Immediate radical resection after local excision of rectal cancer: an oncologic compromise? *Dis Colon Rectum* 2005; **48**: 429–437.

32. Nascimbeni R, Burgart LJ, Nivatvongs S, Larson DR. Risk of lymph node metastasis in T1 carcinoma of the colon and rectum. *Dis Colon Rectum* 2002; **45**: 200–206.

33. Kapiteijn E, Marlinen CAM, Nagtegaal ID *et al.* for the Dutch Rectal Cancer Group. Preoperative radiotherapy combined with total mesorectal excision for resectable cancer. *N Engl J Med* 2001; **345**: 638–646.

34. Cook TA, Mortensen NJMc. Local methods of treatment of rectal cancer. *Colorect Dis* 2000; **2**: 252–263.

35. Winde G, Nottberg H, Keller R, Schmid KW, Bunte H. Surgical cure for early rectal carcinomas (T1). Transanal endoscopic microsurgery versus anterior resection. *Dis Colon Rectum* 1996; **39**: 969–976.

36. Baron PL, Enker WE, Zakowski MF, Urmacher C. Immediate vs. salvage resection after local treatment for early rectal cancer. *Dis Colon Rectum* 1995; **38**: 177–181.

37. Chakravarti A, Compton CC, Shellito PC *et al*. Long-term follow-up of patients with rectal cancer managed by local excision with and without adjuvant irradiation. *Ann Surg* 1999; **230**: 49–54.

38. Lamont JP, McCarthy TM, Digan RD, Jacobson R, Tulanon P, Lichliter WE. Should locally excised T1 rectal cancer receive adjuvant chemoradiation? *Am J Surg* 2000; **180**: 402–406.

39. Garcia-Aquilar J, Mellgren A, Sirivongs P, Buie D, Madoff RD, Rothenberger DA. Local excision of rectal cancer without adjuvant therapy. A word of caution. *Ann Surg* 2000; **231**: 345.

40. Nastro P, Beral D, Hartley J, Monson JRT. Local excision of rectal cancer: review of literature. *Dig Surg* 2005; **22**: 6–15.

41. Zerz A, Muller-Stich BP, Beck J, Linke GR, Tarantino I, Lange J. Endoscopic posterior mesorectal resection after transanal local excision of T1 carcinomas of the lower third of the rectum. *Dis Colon Rectum* 2006; **49**: 919–924.

Sayed Aly John McHale Stephen Barker

12

Stroke and cerebrovertebral reconstruction

In the UK, the incidence of new stroke is 1 in 500; hence, approximately 125,000 new stroke patients present each year. Of these, half are older than 75 years of age and 25% are less than 65 years of age. Stroke management utilises about 10% of all hospital 'bed-available' days and accounts for 5% of annual health care expenditure.[1] With an increasingly ageing population in the UK, as well as across Europe, one might expect an increase in these numbers by some 30% over the next 30 years.[2] Transient ischaemic attacks (TIAs) occur at a rate of 0.5 per 1000 persons. In the US, 500,000 new strokes are reported annually and, at any given time, there are one million stroke victims alive, but disabled. In 1976, the cost of care was estimated at US \$7.5 billion.[3] One can only imagine the cost in 30 years time, with both inflation and an accelerating actual cost of medical care!

CAROTID STENOSIS

The degree of carotid artery stenosis, plaque morphology and plaque progression are known 'risk factors'. Carotid atherosclerotic plaques can be calcified, fibrous, soft or mixed. Calcified plaque is often asymptomatic and soft plaque is often symptomatic. Chambers and Norris[4] reviewed 500 patients

Sayed Aly PhD FRCS (for correspondence)
Consultant Vascular and Endovascular Surgeon, Beaumont/Mater University Hospital, PO 1297, Beaumont Road, Dublin 7, Eire
E-mail: sayed@doctors.org.uk

John McHale MD FAA
Consultant Neuro-anaesthethist, Mater University Hospital, Dublin 7, Eire

Stephen Barker MS FRCS
Senior Lecturer in Surgery and Consultant Vascular Surgeon, University College London, London W1, UK

with neck bruits and a varying degree of stenosis. At one year, TIA or stroke had occurred in 2.1% where the degree of stenosis was less than 30%, in 5.7% with 30–74% stenosis and in 19.5% with 75–100% stenosis. In addition, asymptomatic plaques with a less than 80% stenosis, which later progressed to more than 80%, frequently become symptomatic.[5]

The asymptomatic carotid trial (ACAS) concluded that undertaking surgery was marginally (but significantly) beneficial in patients with more than 60% stenosis (stroke rate 5.1% in the surgical group, compared to 11% in the non-surgical group).[6] The European Carotid Surgery Trial (ECST) and the North American Symptomatic Carotid Endarterectomy Trial (NASCET) produced very similar results. While either medical and surgical management can offer significant benefits, the trials demonstrated the beneficial effect of surgery in those patients with a tight, symptomatic, internal carotid artery stenosis (> 70%). ECST showed that surgery was not indicated in patients with a symptomatic, but minimal, degree of stenosis. With a mild stenosis (50–70%), surgery provide a modest benefit.[7,8]

VERTEBROBASILAR ISCHAEMIA

Because of the frequent uncertainty of the diagnosis of vertebrobasilar ischaemia (VBI), surgery has played a far less prominent role in the management of vertebrobasilar territory TIAs. Data from the Mayo Clinic suggest that the risk of stroke after TIA is similar to that of patients with a similar attack originating from the carotid distribution.[9] Thus, identification of patients who might benefit from surgery is of considerable importance, although identification and treatment of VBI are more difficult than for carotid stenosis.

Key points 1 & 2

- Surgery is indicated in patients with a > 70%, symptomatic, internal carotid artery stenosis.

- Vertebrobasilar ischaemia is difficult to identify and, consequently, is rarely treated

---

PATHOPHYSIOLOGY OF STROKE

ATHEROSCLEROTIC DISEASE

Complications from atherosclerotic lesions (ulceration, or haemorrhage) lead to thrombus formation and thrombus can be dislodged, to pass to the retinal arteries, or to the cerebrum (via the middle cerebral artery), causing a TIA, a complete stroke, amaurosis fugax, or a retinal infarct. VBI is often haemodynamic in origin but a combination of carotid and vertebral artery disease can result in poor perfusion of the hindbrain. 'Steal' syndromes, due to significant disease of the origin of the left subclavian or innominate artery, are another common cause of VBI.

NON-ATHEROSCLEROTIC DISEASES

Abnormal anatomy

Kinks and coiling of carotid vessels are common (and are seen in approximately 20% of patients on angiograms). As a source of embolisation, their clinical significance is debatable. Surgical correction of severe kinking during carotid surgery is important to minimise the risks of postoperative thrombosis.

Fibromuscular dysplasia

This is a rare condition seen in < 1% of patients which affects mainly the renal arteries; some 60% of cases are bilateral, mainly in young women. Four grades are known – intimal and medial fibroplasia, medial hyperplasia and perimedial dysplasia. The majority of patients are asymptomatic. Angioplasty is the treatment of choice in most cases, but some require reconstruction.

Takayasu's arteritis

This is a transmural, granulomatous disease associated with fibrosis and occlusion. It affects mainly young women. In the acute phase, patients present with generalised malaise, fever, myalgia and arthritis. It varies between disease limited to the aortic arch and its branches, to include disease involving the abdominal aorta and the renal vessels. Steroids and cytotoxic agents (cyclophosphamide and methotrexate) are the main-stay of management. If intervention is required, then bypass surgery is preferable as lesions are often long.

Carotid body tumours

These arise from chemoreceptor cells. They are rare (0.012% of resected surgical specimens reported at one hospital).[10] About 10% are bilateral, or multifocal tumours and 10% have a genetic basis. Tumours are benign in 80% and usually occur in patients aged 50–70 years. Local invasion and lymph node metastases, or haematogenous spread, especially to bone, are reported in less than 20%. Other sites of these tumours are in the vagal body, or glomus tumours, or adrenal phaeochromocytomas. A common complaint is of a long-standing lump in the neck but 90% of patients are asymptomatic. Involvement of cranial nerves (VII, IX, X, XI, and XII) results in symptoms such as dysphagia, choking, or hoarseness. Duplex ultrasonography can confirm the diagnosis. Angiography is usually performed if the duplex examination suggests a carotid body tumour, which might demonstrate splaying of the carotid bifurcation and a tumour 'blush'. Enhanced computed tomography is helpful in determining the upper level of a large tumour.

Trauma

Dissection and false aneurysm formation (which cause about 2% of strokes) are complications of trauma. One in five trauma patients who suffer from a neurological deficit have an associated arterial dissection and a quarter of these are found to be bilateral. The majority are symptomatic and ocular signs are common. Duplex ultrasonography can be useful, but an angiogram, or magnetic resonance angiography should be performed. On an angiogram, dissection can be; type 1, where there is intimal irregularity, type 2 when

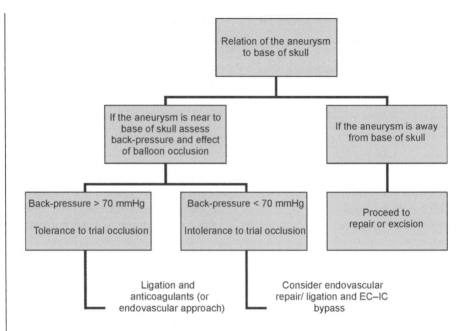

Fig. 1 Management of carotid aneurysm.

associated with stenosis of 70% or more, and type 3, where there is a complete occlusion. Dissection is associated with 30% permanent disability and 20% mortality. Anticoagulants and other conservative treatments are the main-stay of management, but surgery is often best for complicated trauma cases. Follow-up with duplex ultrasonography is required to identify a dissecting aneurysm.

Carotid aneurysm

This represents 4% of all peripheral artery aneurysms. Mostly, patients are asymptomatic until complications such as thrombosis or embolisation occur. Surgery is the treatment of choice, although endovascular options are increasingly feasible (Fig. 1).

CLINICAL PRESENTATION

TIAs are neurological events which last less than 24 h and leave the patient at his or her neurological baseline (Table 1). TIAs in the carotid artery territory reflect its distribution to the eye and the anterior two-thirds of the brain. Weakness, numbness and clumsiness of the limbs, especially the arm, contralateral to the side of the lesion, or loss of vision on the side of the lesion (amaurosis fugax; described as a blind being pulled down, with vision returning, usually within a few minutes) are common symptoms. Dysphasia associated with a TIA is also common, especially if the left hemisphere is involved (in a right-handed person). Global symptoms include faintness, giddiness, vertigo, binocular visual loss and syncope; usually, these are due to a transient fall in blood pressure and, hence, diminished cerebral perfusion. This seldom results in a focal deficit except where there is a tight carotid stenosis.

Table 1 Clinical symptoms associated with carotid disease

- TIA – a neurological event lasting less than 24 h, which leaves the patient at his/her neurological baseline thereafter
- Crescendo TIAs – frequent and recurrent TIAs
- RIND – a reversible, ischaemic, neurological deficit
- Acute stroke/evolving stroke – stroke in progress

The symptoms of VBI can be difficult to recognise. Vertigo and visual loss is a common symptom for one-half fields, to loss on both sides. Bilateral impairment varies from blindness, to a generalised 'mistiness' of vision. Ataxia, diplopia, dysphagia, dysarthria and 'drop attacks' can occur. 'Drop attacks' often occur without loss of consciousness and seem specific to VBI. Furthermore, tingling and numbness of the face and mouth and transient hemiparesis can occur.

Classically, steal syndromes are produced, with exercise of the arm on the appropriate side during clinical examination. This can be associated with a distinct pressure gradient noted between the arms on each side (of at least 20 mmHg). Examination of all systems 'in general' and of the entire vascular system should be performed. Examination of the heart for evidence of valve disease (as a possible source of emboli) is also important. In patients who have had an attack of amaurosis fugax not long before being seen, examination of the fundi may be rewarding in that emboli may still be identified even though vision has recovered. If vision remains defective, an embolus, usually refractile, can often be identified.

Key point 3

- While the diagnosis of carotid artery disease is almost certain, the clinical presentation of vertebrobasilar ischaemia is complex and uncertain.

INVESTIGATIONS

General assessment should include an appraisal of the general condition of the patient and standard blood tests (including an ESR, C-reactive protein, lipid profile, and blood sugar). Careful cardiac evaluation is essential (including an ECG and an echocardiogram), as one-third of patients with carotid TIAs die of a myocardial infarction within 5 years of undergoing carotid endarterectomy.

SPECIFIC INVESTIGATIONS

Intra-arterial digital subtraction angiography
This is necessary to obtain satisfactory pictures (Fig. 2). The risk of a stroke being precipitated by angiography is between 1–4 % (when this is performed for extracerebrovascular assessment).

A 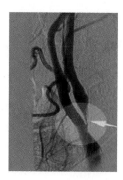 B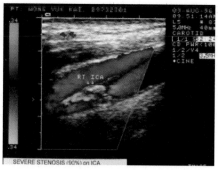

Fig. 2 An internal carotid stenosis is demonstrated on both: (A) intra-arterial digital subtraction angiography (IA DSA); and (B) duplex scanning.

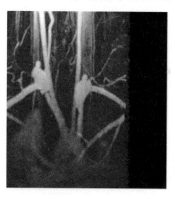

Fig. 3 Magnetic resonance angiography (MRA) scan of a 19-year-old patient involved in a car who presented with cervical injuries associated with bilateral, false vertebro-subclavian aneurysms, with dissection of the left vertebral artery.

Duplex ultrasound scanning

This has accepted accuracy and the degree of stenosis is based on correlating the peak systolic and end-diastolic velocity, with the degree of stenosis as identified on angiography. Image analysis of atherosclerotic plaque also facilitates the differentiation between various types of plaques. Many clinicians have performed carotid endarterectomy based on duplex findings alone.

Magnetic resonance angiography

Magnetic resonance angiography is another form of non-invasive carotid imaging. Carotid magnetic resonance angiography is associated with no known major problems and provides a good and accurate image (Fig. 3).

Transcranial Doppler

Analysis of blood velocity within the intracerebral arteries is a relatively new tool to evaluate cerebral blood flow, but it does have a role in diagnosis.

Key point 4

- Although intra-arterial digital subtraction angiography continues to be the 'gold standard', the accuracy and non-invasive nature of duplex ultrasound scanning provides an acceptable alternative for many clinicians.

MANAGEMENT OF STROKE

In an acute presentation, a patient with a cerebrovascular attack (CVA) or TIA should be assessed and CT and duplex scans should be organised (Fig. 4). These patients will require prompt medical and neurological attention (Table 2). Absolute contra-indications for later carotid endarterectomy are major cerebral infarction, haemorrhage, cerebral oedema and a depressed level of consciousness. If a good response is achieved and providing no contra-indications exist, aspirin 75 mg/day should be given. If a tight stenosis (> 70%) is present, carotid endarterectomy is indicated provided that the patient's general health and, in particular, their cardiac status is sound. Hypertension should be controlled and hyperlipidaemia treated.

In the case of minimal stenosis (0–29%), patients should be maintained on aspirin therapy alone. In the case of a moderate stenosis (30–70%), if TIAs continue to occur during treatment with aspirin, anticoagulation with warfarin, or surgery should be considered.

Table 2 Conditions associated with increased neurological risk following carotid endarterectomy (CEA)

- An active neurological disease process prior to surgery or an urgent procedure
- Hemispheric versus retinal transient ischaemic attack
- Ipsilateral ischaemic lesion on computerised tomography
- Contralateral carotid occlusion
- Impaired consciousness
- Combined CEA and coronary artery bypass graft surgery
- Patients with uncontrolled hypertension, ischaemic heart disease, DM and renal insufficiency

Key point 5

- Conservative medical treatments for acute stroke remain the accepted rule; if a good response is achieved, surgery can be performed at a later stage.

ROLE OF THROMBOLYSIS IN ACUTE STROKE

The extremely small 'time-window' for treatment and very low recanalisation rates (in the range of 50–65%) in large artery strokes are the major shortcomings of thrombolysis. In 45 patients who were treated with i.v. recombinant tissue plasminogen activator (rt-PA),[11] initial CT angiography showed relevant

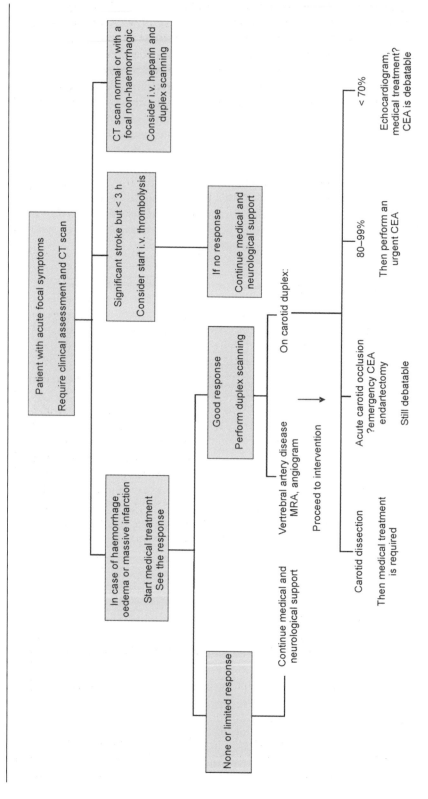

Fig. 4 Acute presentation of cerebrovascular attack (CVA).

arterial occlusions in 35 patients.[11] Recanalisation after rt-PA therapy was demonstrated by digital subtraction angiography in only seven of the 31 patients. At present, there are two major randomised controlled trials sponsored by the National Institutes of Health to test endovascular treatments in acute stroke. Better outcome of endovascular treatment is achieved when a good perfusion effect of the brain tissues is detected on MRI scan and associated with a minimal diffusion or no diffusion abnormality[12] (perfusion/ diffusion ratio).

Key point 6

- A multimodal treatment strategy is often employed to achieve rapid recanalisation of occluded cerebral vessels and to minimise chances of haemorrhage. This may become the standard of care in the future.

ANAESTHESIA FOR CAROTID SURGERY

The goals of intra-operative anaesthetic management for carotid endarterectomy are: (i) prevention of cerebral and myocardial ischaemia; (ii) maintenance of haemodynamic stability; and (iii) rapid recovery of the patient to allow a prompt evaluation of their neurological function. While some patients may require general anaesthesia, endarterectomy can often be performed under local anaesthesia (Table 3).

Neurological testing, during carotid endarterectomy performed under regional anaesthesia, is a sensitive marker of cerebral function and can reveal clinically significant cerebral ischaemia even when sensitive EEG monitoring remains unchanged. A reduced 'stump' pressure is associated with a higher risk of ischaemic changes on EEG, but it is neither a specific nor sensitive guide to the use of selective carotid shunting. Transcranial Doppler ultrasonography may be helpful in differentiating between intra-operative, haemodynamic versus embolic, neurological events. Somatosensory-evoked potentials may be useful in the assessment of sub-cortical ischaemia. Near-infrared spectroscopy assesses changes in cerebral blood flow by measuring regional cerebral oxygenation (rSO_2). Questions remain about the precise role of near-infra red spectroscopy compared with other monitors of cerebral ischaemia.[13,14]

Table 3 Disadvantages of regional anaesthesia

- The operation may be technically more difficult, which may increase the risk of an adverse outcome
- Patients may have pain and subsequently, increases the risk of myocardial infarction
- It is unsuitable for those cases which are technically very difficult
- Some patients will refuse to undergo the operation while awake and some surgeons will refuse to perform CEA under regional anaesthesia

A superficial and/or deep cervical plexus block, cervical epidural block, local infiltration, or a combination of these techniques have all been used successfully.

A superficial cervical plexus block is performed with the patient in the supine position and the head turned to the side opposite to the block. A line is drawn from the mastoid process to Chassaignac's tubercle on the C6 transverse process. The needle is inserted over the transverse process of C2. Once bone is encountered, the needle is pulled back slightly. After negative aspiration, 5 ml of local anaesthetic is injected slowly. This is repeated at the other two transverse processes. Local anaesthetic supplementation by the surgeon will usually be required, especially if a high carotid lesion requires aggressive retraction on the mandible.

Key point 7

- Carotid endarterectomy can be done under either general or regional anaesthesia.

CAROTID ENDARTERECTOMY

The carotid bifurcation is exposed along the anterior border of the sternomastoid muscle. Having exposed the carotid bifurcation, the common carotid artery (CCA) is clamped and the internal carotid (ICA) 'back-pressure' is recorded as a 'stump pressure'. It is a measure of the collateral flow from the other side of the head and the vertebrobasilar system, via the circle of Willis. Surgeons who shunt selectively would consider pressure below 50–60 mmHg an indication for a shunt to be placed. The patient is heparinised and clamps are applied. An arteriotomy, starting in the common carotid artery, below the lesion, is carried through the lesion in to the internal carotid artery, distal to the disease. It is essential to obtain a tightly adherent distal flap in the internal carotid artery; if this is not the case, it should be tacked down. Patching is used (with a vein, polytetrafluoroethylene, or Dacron patch) as a means to prevent a recurrent stenosis. Postoperatively, it is important to maintain a stable blood pressure. If any neurological deficit appears, relevant to the side of operation in the early postoperative period, a rapid return to the operating room is indicated, with exploration of the neck and further exposure of the carotid vessels. In the late postoperative period, CT of the brain and duplex scan are required. Re-exploration and a careful inspection of the distal flap site are mandatory. If thrombosis and occlusion of the internal carotid artery have occurred, restoration of the cerebral flow may increase the likelihood of recovery, or at least, limit the extent of the neurological deficit.

Key point 8

- Postoperatively, it is important to maintain a stable blood pressure. If a neurological deficit appears, a rapid return to the operating room is indicated.

Table 4 The Shamblin classification of carotid body tumours

Grade	Criteria	Cases
Group 1	Easy to remove from the vessels	25%
Group 2	Requires dissection in a sub-adventitial plane to remove them from the vessel	50%
Group 3	The tumour encircles and invades the vessel to such an extent that it usually requires complete arterial excision and replacement with a length of saphenous vein	25%

CAROTID BODY TUMOURS

Factors that influence the operative decision are tumour size and tumour involvement of adjacent structures, together with a slow rate of growth (Table 4).

If tumours are deemed benign, their natural course is of slow enlargement, with eventual compression of local structures resulting in symptoms such as nerve palsy. In the elderly patient without symptoms, it may be appropriate to do nothing. However, it is much easier and safer to remove the tumour before extensive local invasion occurs and so, in most patients, a surgical approach is advised when the tumour is still small. Untreated, 75% of asymptomatic patients eventually develop symptoms and 30% will die from invasion of local structures or from metastatic disease.

In large (> 3 cm) and very vascular tumours, embolisation can be used to minimise excessive surgical blood loss. There are usually communications between the main feeding vessels of the tumour from the external carotid artery and the vertebral artery; embolisation via the external carotid may result in embolisation to the brain. It is important to assess cranial nerve involvement, but it is useful also to look for invasion of the pharynx by upward extension of the tumour (which is a rare occurrence). CT and MRI are required to assess the upward extension of the tumour and to determine any invasion at the skull base. Magnetic resonance angiography, may provide some advantages over CT as the soft tissue contrast is probably better in determining the extent of invasion by a large tumour. Its greater sensitivity allows detection of tumours down to 5 mm in diameter.[15,16]

Operation

Experience with carotid artery surgery is important (Fig. 5). The carotid arteries are each exposed and are controlled beyond the tumour. Some surgeons divide, or at least clamp, the external carotid near its origin, as soon as possible to reduce the vascularity of the tumour and improve access. The Connell technique, in which a straight shunt is inserted via the common carotid into the internal carotid, is effective at devascularising the tumour. The dissection should start at the bifurcation and the tumour should be rolled upwards early on, to get a clear view of the cranial nerves. Misdiagnosis of a vagal body tumour has been reported, which arises very close to the carotid bifurcation and can be easily mistaken for the former. The vagus nerve itself is

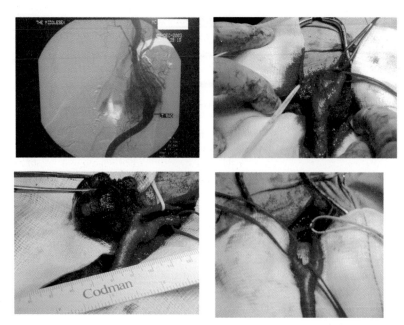

Fig. 5 Carotid body tumour in a 49-year-old woman who presented with a painless slow growing neck lump. On the angiography a vascular tumour was identified. The lump was wrapped around the CCA and ECA and was successfully excised.

involved and, therefore, has to be sacrificed. If a carotid body tumour extends well up into the neck, deliberate fracture of the styloid process can improve access. It may be necessary to dislocate forward the temporomandibular joint, to gain access to its upper border.

Cranial nerve damage is reported in 10–20% of cases, although most recover within a few weeks. Bilateral carotid body tumours should not be removed simultaneously.

In patients who have had surgery to a previous carotid body tumour resulting in cranial nerve palsy, or carotid occlusion, the risks of operation on a contralateral tumour are considerable and radiotherapy (see below) may be preferable. Cerebrovascular accidents occur in less than 3% of cases, in most series.

Radiotherapy
Most centres recommend surgery as the best treatment of choice, while radiotherapy is used only for tumours too extensive to excise, or as a backup treatment for those with recurrence. Most patients are cured by surgery and cranial nerve palsies are usually temporary. A few patients prove to have a malignant tumour, noted because of local invasion or metastatic disease. Local

Key point 9
- Surgery is the accepted treatment for small carotid body tumours, with embolisation reserved for large tumours. Radiotherapy has a limited role as a primary treatment. Large, asymptomatic tumours in unfit patients require no treatment.

radiotherapy can be used to prevent local recurrence, or to treat metastatic disease. Carotid body tumours are thought to be somewhat radioresistant. In summary, 23% showed a complete response, 54% a partial response and 23% no response.[17,18] Most tumours are slow growing and survival for many years is possible even with established metastatic disease.

CAROTID ANEURYSM

Carotid aneurysm is a rare condition. Presentation is usually 'incidental'. A complication in the form of a thrombosis or embolisation is reported, but rupture is rare. The initial diagnosis is established on duplex or magnetic resonance angiography scanning. Selective angiography is required to establish the extent of the aneurysm and its relation to other vessels. Also, during the angiogram, measurement of the internal carotid artery 'stump' pressure while occluding distally with a balloon and the period of temporary carotid occlusion should be recorded. Determination of relation to the base of skull is essential (Fig. 1).

Key point 10
- Management of carotid aneurysm depends on distance from the base of skull.

SURGERY FOR VERTEBRAL ARTERY DISEASE

The vertebral arteries originate from the first part of the subclavian artery. The vertebral artery (VA) consists of four parts.

V1 The artery runs upward and backward, behind the internal jugular and vertebral veins. The left VA is crossed by the thoracic duct. Exploration of V1 is through a transverse supraclavicular incision in the root of the neck. Division of the sternomastoid muscle is usually required. A stenosis of the origin of VA may be approached directly. The artery can be divided distal to the lesion and re-implanted in to the CCA. Alternatively, an endarterectomy is performed at the origin or preferably, through the subclavian artery.

V2 The artery then runs upward through the foramina in the transverse processes of the upper six cervical vertebrae and pursues an almost vertical course as far as the transverse process of the atlas. A direct approach is required only in the case of trauma; otherwise, bypass surgery is more appropriate.

V3 V3 issues from the last foramen on the medial side of the rectus capitis lateralis and curves backwards, behind the superior articular process of the atlas (the anterior ramus of the first cervical nerve being on its medial side). It then lies in the groove on the upper surface of the posterior arch of the atlas and enters the vertebral canal by passing

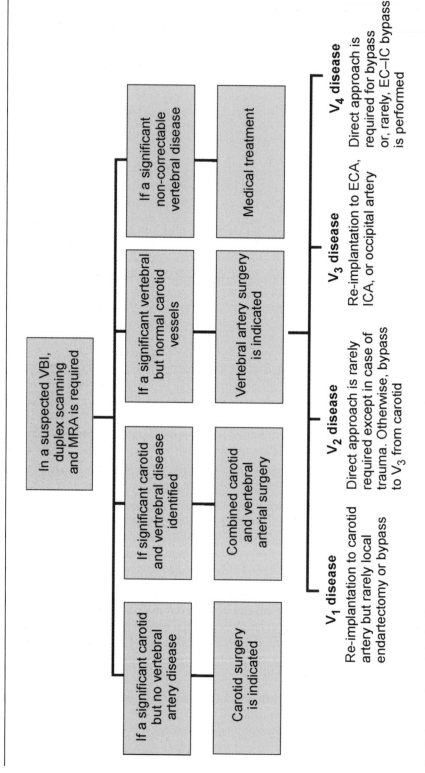

Fig. 6 Surgery for vertebrobasilar system.

beneath the posterior atlanto-occipital membrane and is contained in the sub-occipital triangle. Through a high pre-sternomastotid incision, this part is accessible. Re-implantation of V3, to the ECA, or ICA, or occipital artery is required.

V4 The artery pierces the dura mater and inclines medially to the front of the medulla oblongata. It is placed between the hypoglossal nerve and the anterior root of the first cervical nerve and beneath the first digitation of the ligamentum denticulatum. At the lower border of the pons, the VA unites with the vessel from the opposite side to form the basilar artery. A direct approach from the occipital triangle is required. Reports of using EC–IC bypass demonstrate the feasibility of the reconstruction.

Steal syndromes
In subclavian steal, when an endovascular option fails, a prosthetic graft or vein is inserted 'end-to-side' between the common carotid artery and the subclavian artery, distal to the origin of the vertebral artery. Alternatively, an axillary–axillary bypass can be used. With innominate steal, the simplest approach is to implant a Dacron graft from the arch of the aorta to the distal innominate artery at its bifurcation. The innominate artery and its origin from the arch of the aorta are best approached via a median sternotomy.

Results of surgery
Surgery for VBI, which now rarely involves opening the chest, can be performed with minimal morbidity (Fig. 6). However, it is much more difficult to evaluate the efficacy of surgery in terms of relief of symptoms, because of the varied nature of the symptom complex. Nevertheless, with careful selection of patients, the outcome can be favourable. The outcome of surgery for innominate, or subclavian artery steals in terms of symptom relief is much better in general, than for vertebral artery surgery. If severe bilateral carotid stenoses are present, in a patient with symptoms of vertebrobasilar ischaemia, the most appropriate procedure might well be a carotid endarterectomy.[19,20]

Endovascular management
Carotid stenting is a relatively new and controversial treatment for carotid artery disease. Progress now is mainly with cerebral protection devices and less with direct development of catheter and delivery systems. Universally accepted indications for such treatment are when surgery is deemed either difficult or impossible, without high risk of complications, for example in high or recurrent disease and in the case of previous neck irradiation. The trans-femoral approach tends to be used. Several protection devices are available (see examples in Fig. 7), although complications are reported. Using a stent as a primary treatment is a major area of controversy, since carotid surgery is associated with such a low rate of complications.[21]

CONCLUSIONS

Stroke is not a common medical disorder. It has an impact on not only the patient, but also on society and the entire health service. Stroke has to be

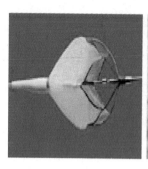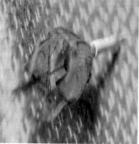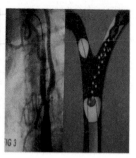

Fig. 7 Types of the neuroprotection devices: 'spider' and reverse flow (MOMA).

prevented by all means (screening, medical and surgical management) and, in addition, researchers should be encouraged to identify the responsible factors which lead to instability of carotid plaques. More studies are required to assess the actual indications of simultaneous carotid–coronary artery surgery in asymptomatic patients. Carotid endarterectomy has proved to be safe over the last 50 years and benefits most patients in both the short- and the long-term, while most of the reports concerning carotid stents remain uncertain about both the indications and long-term outcome (Table 5). Most authors believe that carotid stents should be reserved for difficult cases (such as high lesions and recurrent symptomatic disease) until we obtain clear evidence that it safe to be used as primary treatment for carotid artery disease. VBI requires a close co-operation with neurologists before embarking on any management strategy.

Table 5 Complications of carotid endarterectomy (CEA)

- The major complications of CEA are death, either from stroke or a myocardial infarction
- The combined peri-operative mortality and major stroke rate should be less than 5%
- A neurological deficit may be due to thrombosis at the site of endarterectomy, with either occlusion or embolisation, or with an intracerebral haemorrhage
- As most patients will be receiving aspirin, significant haematomas are relatively common, but rarely need draining
- Local nerve pareses are not uncommon, but are usually transient, recovering within weeks to months. In the case of the hypoglossal nerve and a high carotid bifurcation, retraction is the usual cause of local nerve paresis, which is often unavoidable. Retraction of the vagus may result in paresis of the superior or recurrent laryngeal nerves
- Re-stenosis: availability of duplex ultrasound scanning has shown that the incidence of recurrent stenosis is 15–30% at 5 years. However, symptoms are very uncommon

Key points for clinical practice

- Surgery is indicated in patients with a > 70%, symptomatic, internal carotid artery stenosis.

- Vertebrobasilar ischaemia is difficult to identify and, consequently, is rarely treated.

- While the diagnosis of carotid artery disease is almost certain, the clinical presentation of vertebrobasilar ischaemia is complex and uncertain.

- Although intra-arterial digital subtraction angiography continues to be the 'gold standard', the accuracy and non-invasive nature of duplex ultrasound scanning provides an acceptable alternative for many clinicians.

- Conservative medical treatments for acute stroke remain the accepted rule; if a good response is achieved, surgery can be performed at a later stage.

- A multimodal treatment strategy is often employed to achieve rapid recanalisation of occluded cerebral vessels and to minimise chances of haemorrhage. This may become the standard of care in the future.

- Carotid endarterectomy can be done under either general or regional anaesthesia.

- Postoperatively, it is important to maintain a stable blood pressure. If a neurological deficit appears, a rapid return to the operating room is indicated.

- Surgery is the accepted treatment for small carotid body tumours, with embolisation reserved for large tumours. Radiotherapy has a limited role as a primary treatment. Large, asymptomatic tumours in unfit patients require no treatment.

- Management of carotid aneurysm depends on distance from the base of skull.

References

1. McGuire AJ, Raikou M, Whittle I, Christensen MC. Long-term mortality, morbidity and hospital care following intracerebral haemorrhage: an 11-year cohort study. *Cerebrovasc Dis* 2007; **23**: 221–228.
2. Lee WC, Christensen MC, Joshi AV, Pashos CL. Long-term cost of stroke subtypes among Medicare beneficiaries *Cerebrovasc Dis* 2007; **23**: 57–65.
3. Brown DL, Boden-Albala B, Langa KM *et al*. Projected costs of ischemic stroke in the United States. *Neurology* 2006; **67**: 1390–1395.
4. Chambers BR, Norris JW. Outcome in patients with asymptomatic neck bruits. *N Engl J Med* 1986; **315**: 860–865.
5. Norris JW, Zhu CZ, Bornstein NM, Chambers BR. Vascular risks of asymptomatic carotid stenosis. *Stroke* 1991; **22**: 1485–1490.
6. Young B, Moore WS, Robertson JT *et al*. An analysis of perioperative surgial mortality and morbidity in the asymptomatic carotid Artherosclerosis Study. ACAS Investigators. Asymptomatic Carotid Atherosclerosis Study. *Stroke* 1996; **27**: 2216–2224.

7. European Carotid Surgery Trialist's Collaborative Group (1991). MRC European Carotid Surgery Trial: interim results for symptomatic patients with severe or with mild carotid stenosis. *Lancet* 1991; **337**: 1235–1243.

8. North American Symptomatic Carotid Endarterectomy Trial Collaborators. Beneficial effect of carotid endarterectomy in symptomatic patients with high-grade carotid stenosis. *N Engl J Med* 1991; **325**: 445–453.

9. Cartlidge NE, Whisnant JP, Elveback LR. Carotid and vertebral-basilar transient cerebral ischemic attacks. A community study, Rochester, Minnesota. *Mayo Clin Proc* 1977; **52**: 117–120.

10. Hallett Jr JW, Nora JD, Hollier LH, Cherry Jr KJ, Pairolero PC. Trends in neurovascular complications of surgical management for carotid body and cervical paragangliomas: a fifty-year experience with 153 tumors. *J Vasc Surg* 1988; **7**: 284–291.

11. Lee KY, Han SW, Kim SH *et al*. Early recanalization after intravenous administration of recombinant tissue plasminogen activator as assessed by pre- and post-thrombolytic angiography in acute ischemic stroke patients. *Stroke* 2007; **38**: 192–193.

12. Edgell R, Yavagal DR. Acute endovascular stroke therapy. *Curr Neurol Neurosci Report* 2006; **6**: 531–538.

13. McCrory DC, Goldstein LB, Samsa GP *et al*. Predicting complications of carotid endarterectomy. *Stroke* 1993; **24**: 1285–1291.

14. Goldstein LB, McCrory DC, Landsman PB *et al*. Multicenter review of preoperative risk factors for carotid endarterectomy in patients with ipsilateral symptoms. *Stroke* 1994; **25**: 1116–1121.

15. McPherson GA, Halliday AW, Mansfield AO. Carotid body tumours and other cervical paragangliomas: diagnosis and management in 25 patients. *Br J Surg* 1989; **76**: 33–36.

16. LaMuraglia GM, Fabian RL, Brewster DC *et al*. The current surgical management of carotid body paragangliomas. *J Vasc Surg* 1992; **15**: 1038–1045.

17. Evenson LJ, Mendenhall WM, Pearsons JT, Cassisi NJ. Radiotherapy in the management of the carotid body and glomus vagale. *Head Neck* 1998; **20**: 609–613.

18. Hinerman RW, Mendenhall WM, Amdur RJ, Stringer SP, Antonelli PJ, Cassisi NJ. Definitive radiotherapy in the management of chemodectomas arising in the temporal bone, carotid body and glomus vagale. *Head Neck* 2001; **23**: 363–371.

19. Regli L, Piepgras DG, Hansen KK. Late patency of long saphenous vein by-pass grafts to the anterior and posterior cerebral. *Circ J Neurosurg* 1995; **83**: 806–811.

20. Morris PJ. Surgery of vertebrobasilar disease. In: Warlow C, Morris PJ. (eds) *Transient Ischemic Attacks*. New York: Marcel Dekker, 1982; 297.

21. Mas JL, Chatellier G, Beyssen B *et al*. EVA-3S Investigators. Endarterectomy versus stenting in patients with symptomatic severe carotid stenosis. *N Engl J Med* 2006; **355**: 1660–1671.

Fiona McCaig   Udi Chetty

13

Sentinel node biopsy and axillary surgery in breast surgery

The management of the axilla in patients with breast cancer remains controversial. During the period when radical surgery was performed for all patients with breast cancer, the aim was to remove the breast and all the draining lymph nodes in the axilla and, in some cases, the internal mammary chain. This radical approach was associated with considerable morbidity and, in randomised clinical trials, showed no survival advantage over less radical surgery.[1] More recently, with the realisation that there is a spectrum of breast cancers with varying potential to spread, a tailored approach to the management of the axilla has developed. Table 1 illustrates the variation in axillary node involvement related to the grade and size of tumour, which shows the range from 14% to 60% of node involvement.[2] Evidence is emerging that the molecular pathology of tumours will add further to the ability to predict whether the lymph nodes are involved.

In this modern era, the aim is to determine whether the nodes are involved or not. Axillary nodal involvement is considered to be the single most important prognostic indicator in women with breast cancer. If the nodes are not involved, no treatment to the axilla is required. If the nodes are involved, an axillary clearance or radiotherapy should be undertaken. Establishing lymph node involvement pre-operatively is useful as it may avert the need for further surgery. The overall aim is to reduce the chance of disease recurrence with the minimum degree of morbidity.

Fiona McCaig BSc(Hons) MBChB
Research Fellow, Edinburgh Breast Unit, Western General Hospital, Crewe Road, Edinburgh EH4 2XU, UK. E-mail: fionamccaig@doctors.org.uk

Udi Chetty BSc ChB FRCS MRCP (for correspondence)
Consultant Surgeon, Edinburgh Breast Unit, Western General Hospital, Crewe Road, Edinburgh EH4 2XU, UK. E-mail: udi.chetty@luht.scot.nhs.uk

ANATOMY AND LYMPHATIC DRAINAGE OF THE BREAST

There are approximately 20–25 lymph nodes in the fibrofatty tissue of the axilla as shown in Figure 1. For surgical purposes, this pyramidal compartment can be divided into three levels depending on their relationship with the pectoralis

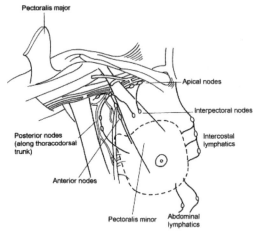

Fig. 1 The principal lymphatic drainage of the breast is to the axilla which includes the anterior, posterior and apical nodes.

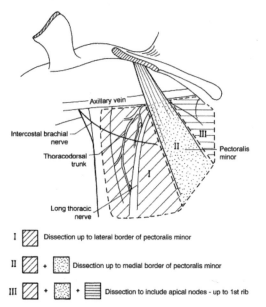

Fig. 2 Axillary levels for lymph node sampling. The axilla can be divided into levels I, II and III, depending on their relationship to the pectoralis minor muscle.

Table 1 The incidence of axillary metastatic disease for invasive ductal breast cancer

Size of tumour	Tumour grade		
(mm)	Grade I	Grade II	Grade III
1–10	14%	15%	40%
11–20	24%	34%	51%
21–50	29%	42%	60%

minor muscle, as shown in Figure 2. Level I contains approximately 15 nodes and, by definition, lies below and lateral to the inferolateral border of the pectoralis minor muscle. Level II contains 4 or 5 nodes and is located posterior to the pectoralis minor muscle. There are usually only 2 or 3 nodes located in level III which lie superior to the upper border of the pectoralis minor.

Lymph node involvement by tumour cells tends to be progressive from levels I to III. Skip involvement of nodes (*i.e.* where a higher echelon node is involved when the lower echelon node is uninvolved) is unusual and has been demonstrated to occur in <5% of patients.[3] An isolated axillary node metastasis at level III does not 'skip' levels I and II, but instead represents a site of direct lymphatic drainage.[4] The breast also drains to interpectoral and internal mammary nodes.

Key point 2

- In > 95% of breast cancers, cells metastasise to the axilla in a progressive manner from levels I to III.[3]

METHODS TO DETERMINE WHETHER LYMPH NODES ARE INVOLVED

NON-OPERATIVE STAGING

Clinical examination

Clinical examination of the axilla has been shown to be inaccurate in determining nodal involvement, with an overall sensitivity and specificity of between 50–70%. If there are enlarged and palpable nodes, cytology obtained by fine needle aspiration or histology obtained by core biopsy can provide a definitive diagnosis. Large lymph nodes do not necessarily represent metastatic disease and involved nodes are often impalpable. Nodes can become enlarged for several reasons (*e.g.* reactive nodes secondary to inflammation or the procedure of core biopsy).

Key point 3

- Clinical examination of the axilla is 50–70% reliable in identifying metastatic lymph nodes.

Mammography

Mammography is a sensitive method of detecting large axillary lymph nodes but has a low specificity.

Ultrasonography with or without fine needle aspiration or core biopsy

Pre-operative ultrasonography is being used increasingly to assess and stage the axilla in women with breast cancer. This method can potentially identify between 40–50% of node-positive patients and identify those patients who require an axillary clearance.[5] Nodes that show abnormal morphology should be further assessed by fine needle aspiration or core biopsy. Ultrasonography-guided fine needle aspiration is a simple, minimally invasive, easily available technique which has been reported to have a sensitivity of 97.4% and specificity of 79.9% in a recent study.[6] Axillary ultrasonography with guided fine needle aspiration of abnormal nodes allows pre-operative diagnosis of nodal status in a third of screen-detected and approaching a half of symptomatic breast cancer patients.[6] Those who have a positive fine needle aspiration or core biopsy should proceed to axillary lymph node dissection whilst those who show no evidence of involvement may undergo sentinel node biopsy/axillary sampling. It is now our routine practice to have an ultrasound assessment of the axillary nodes in all patients with invasive breast cancer. It should be noted, however, that the accuracy of axillary ultrasonography depends on the experience of the operator.

PET/MRI

Positive emission tomography (PET) is a non-invasive method of staging the axilla and involves the intravenous administration of a positron-labelled metabolic substrate which selectively accumulates in tumour cells compared to normal cells. [18]Fluoro-2-deoxy-D-glucose is the radio-pharmaceutical agent commonly used and its differential uptake is demonstrated using a PET scanner. This technique is developing rapidly; however, it is expensive and not widely available. It is not yet a practical proposition for all clinics but its results are promising, showing a sensitivity of 75% and a specificity of 90% in recent studies. The ability of current PET technology to detect low-volume nodal disease requires improvement.

Magnetic resonance imaging (MRI) remains a problem-solving tool in breast imaging (*e.g.* to evaluate breasts with implants, detect recurrence and assess the breasts of patients with involved axillary nodes). It can demonstrate axillary metastatic disease, but its sensitivity is not sufficient for it to replace surgical staging of the axilla.

OPERATIVE STAGING

Surgical staging of the axilla remains the gold standard. There are several operative procedures that can be undertaken to gain information regarding the status of axillary nodes. These include sentinel lymph node biopsy, axillary sampling, a combination of these two techniques, and finally axillary lymph node dissection, also known as axillary clearance.

Sentinel lymph node biopsy

The term sentinel originates from the Italian word *sentinella* which refers to a guard whose job is to stand and keep watch. The concept of the sentinel node is that tumour drains via lymphatic channels to the regional lymph nodes. The first node in the pathway is the sentinel node; if this is not involved by tumour, the remaining lymph nodes in that drainage basin should be clear of malignancy. This is demonstrated in Figure 3A. The conventional method of identifying the sentinel node involves a dual localisation technique (*i.e.* injecting a radiolabelled colloid and blue dye around the tumour which is then followed by surgical exploration of the axilla). The sentinel node is identified using a hand-held gamma probe detecting a radioactivity count greater than 10 times the background count (usually measured on the arm) and visually by blue staining of the nodes. Sentinel nodes may be hot and blue, hot and non-blue or blue and cold.[7] In practice, rather than a single sentinel node, the average number of sentinel nodes found is 2.9.[8] This could be because there is more than one channel draining the tumour, labelling at least two nodes as shown in Figure 3B. Alternatively, a first and second level/echelon node may be stained, as illustrated in Figure 3C. A false negative result (3.6%[9]) is occasionally due to tumour blocking the lymphatic channels and, therefore, the dye and colloid cannot drain to the sentinel node, but could stain other nodes via alternative pathways. Such 'skip' nodes are shown in Figure 4.

The standard method of performing a sentinel node biopsy is to inject the radiolabelled colloid (technetium-labelled albumin or sulphur colloid) into the breast parenchyma, approximately 2 h prior to the procedure. Lymphoscintigraphy is then usually performed, providing a map of lymphatic drainage. The sentinel node is demonstrated, as is the presence of multiple sentinel nodes and further locations (*e.g.* internal mammary nodes). Blue dye (isosulphane blue, patent blue V or methylene blue) is injected around the tumour, about 15 min prior to the

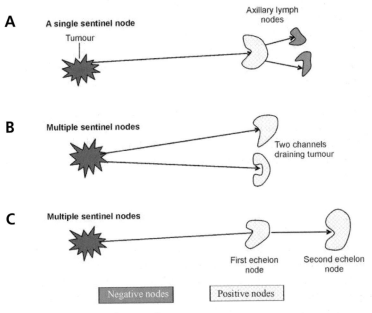

Fig. 3 Pattern of metastatic spread.

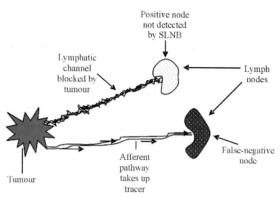

Positive node
not detected
by SLNB

Lymphatic
channel
blocked by
tumour

Lymph
nodes

False-negative
node

Afferent
pathway
takes up
tracer

Tumour

Fig. 4 Lymphatic drainage blocked by tumour leading to a false-negative sentinel node.

operation, usually in the anaesthetic room. The site for injection of colloid and dye varies between centres and there are several different possible locations which will be discussed. A skin crease incision is then made and the sentinel node(s) is identified using a combination of gamma-ray detection using a probe wrapped in a sterile glove and visually identifying any blue-stained nodes. These nodes are excised and subsequently examined for the presence of tumour cells.

Drainage to the internal mammary nodes is demonstrated on lympho-scintigraphy in 9% of cases[8,9] and is better illustrated using peritumoural injection.[10] Inner quadrant location of tumours are most commonly associated with internal mammary node involvement (74%).[11] To biopsy the internal mammary sentinel node requires exploration of the relevant intercostal space medially by dividing the intercostal muscle, carefully avoiding opening the pleural cavity. These nodes are encapsulated in fat and surround the internal mammary vessels. Great care is, therefore, required for successful dissection and preservation of haemostasis. Once identified, the blue/hot node is excised. The procedure can be technically demanding and is prone to cause pneumothorax. The finding of a negative axilla and positive extra-axillary nodes is rare; therefore, the added value of excising extra-axillary lymph nodes is debatable. Internal mammary node positivity is, however, related to a worse prognosis and, once proven, should prompt further local and systemic treatment. One could argue that without internal mammary node sampling, patients may be understaged, resulting in inadequate treatment. Positive internal mammary nodes require irradiation of the internal mammary nodes chain and infra- or supraclavicular nodes. There is currently no data available concerning the advantage of extra-axillary staging and most clinicians do not recommend the routine removal of lymphoscintigraphically positive extra-axillary lymph nodes as the reduction of morbidity is the main goal of sentinel node biopsy.[10]

Key point 4

- Removal of extra-axillary sentinel lymph nodes such as the internal mammary node is not routinely carried out.

If axillary sentinel nodes are found to be infiltrated by tumour, then the patient should undergo axillary lymph node dissection or radiotherapy. The axilla is often irradiated with the supraclavicular fossae to control regional disease. Radiotherapy fields should include the internal mammary nodes for medial tumours or where the internal mammary nodes are likely to be involved.

The sentinel lymph node biopsy technique confers certain advantages for node-negative patients. There is less upper limb morbidity (only a few cases of lymphoedema have been reported in the literature[12]) compared to axillary clearance, and there is improved quality of life as seen by the results of the ALMANAC study.[8] Sentinel lymph node biopsy is an elegant procedure which is associated with a reduction in theatre time and hospital stay. However, it has limitations. Obese women and those with tumours located in areas other than the upper outer quadrant are more likely to have failed localisation of the sentinel lymph node.[13]

Sentinel lymph node biopsy is expensive and requires access to nuclear physics' facilities which may not be possible in smaller institutions. If the sentinel lymph node is positive, then a further operation may be required if intra-operative lymph node assessment is not available. Delayed assessment of the sentinel lymph node biopsy with haematoxylin and eosin (H&E) staining results in 25–30% of patients with sentinel node metastases needing further axillary surgery at a later date.[14] Further surgery can be avoided if frozen sections or imprint cytology is performed intra-operatively, enabling an immediate decision to whether axillary lymph node dissection is warranted. This requires the input of pathologists and is expensive. The adoption of intra-operative sentinel lymph node biopsy using real-time qualitative polymerase chain reaction (PCR) technology (now commercially available: GeneSearch™ Breast Lymph Node Assay, Viridex) has shown promising results, improving patient outcomes and also being cost-efficient. Large-scale, multicentre clinical studies are currently underway to validate One-Step Nucleic Acid Amplification (OSNA) which is another promising alternative to conventional methods, using rapid molecular analysis of sentinel lymph node biopsy material. So far, it has provided rapid results comparable to histological investigation, preventing diagnostic delay and, hence, further surgery.[15] Gene expression profiling from blood may prove a useful determinant of lymph node status on breast cancer patients in the future.

Modification of the standard technique

Lymphatic drainage from the dermis and sub-dermal layer is 5 times greater than from the breast parenchyma. The tracer material may be injected peritumourally, intradermally or in the peri- and sub-areolar region pre-operatively, 10–15 min prior to surgery followed by gentle massage of the breast. Injecting into the sub-areolar space in the segment of the tumour has been shown to be an effective way of identifying the lymph nodes,[16] and is now widely practiced. However, a recent paper from Cambridge suggests that injection into the breast parenchyma may more accurately represent the drainage of the tumour.[16]

> ## Key point 5
> - Injecting blue dye and radioactive tracer in the sub-areolar space in the segment of the tumour is an effective way of identifying the sentinel lymph node.

Which dye to use?

1. **Isosulphane blue** – Isosulphane blue (Lymphazurin) is an aniline dye and is an isomer of patent blue dye. It is widely used in the US, though a few centres, having experienced serious side-effects (anaphylactic reactions in 1.6% of patients[17]), have changed to using methylene blue (methylthioninium chloride).

2. **Methylene blue** – The staining of nodes with methylene blue is not as bright; therefore, the nodes can be harder to find. There have, however, been no severe allergic reactions reported in the literature.[17]

3. **Patent Blue V** – In Europe, patent blue V is widely used and it is estimated that a mild adverse reaction occurs in 1 in 200 patients. Reactions range from blue hives, urticaria, rash and pruritus through to anaphylaxis. There have been 0.25 cases of severe anaphylactic reaction per 10,000 vials sold (Aspen Pharmacare, St Leonards, NSW, Australia).[18] This is probably a considerable underestimate as it only takes into account the numbers reported in the literature or to the company.

There are no studies comparing theses agents directly.

The need for pre-operative lymphoscintigraphy

Pre-operative lymphoscintigraphy provides a map of the lymphatic drainage, demonstrating the exact site and number of sentinel lymph nodes including any aberrant locations. It is useful in the training period when learning the sentinel lymph node technique and if the aim is to determine internal mammary node involvement.

Following injection, sequential images using a gamma camera are obtained at regular intervals, until the initial draining node(s) is visualised. The procedure usually takes 15–35 min, demands that the patient is immobile throughout and requires a nuclear medicine department. All studies have reported an improved detection rate of the sentinel lymph node when combining pre-operative lymphoscintigraphy, intra-operative gamma detection and blue dye together. A recent study showed that visualisation of an axillary sentinel lymph node using pre-operative lymphoscintigraphy was associated with a 98.7% detection rate compared to 93% without pre-operative lymphoscintigraphy.[19] Despite recommendations, this technique is not absolutely necessary and there are a number of surgeons who consider it complex, offering no real additional benefit. However, it is recommended when sentinel lymph node surgery is being carried out by less experienced teams. The hand-held Compact Peri-Operative Imager (POCI) is currently being evaluated as an alternative.[20]

The need for two tracers

Several multicentre studies have shown that combining blue dye and radiolabelled colloid results in improved sentinel lymph node detection rates. Currently, dual labelling is recommended as it improves detection rates and reduces the number of false-negatives (either 92% versus both 95%).[21]

Combining node sampling with the sentinel node biopsy technique

The node sampling technique involves an intra-operative digital examination of the axillary lymph nodes starting at the axillary tail, working upwards and removing at least four lymph nodes. In two large clinical trials,[22,23] comparing a node sample to clearance of the lymph nodes, the positivity rate was similar. The limitation of this technique is that it is not guided and very operator dependent. The blue dye assisted node sampling process is being used as routine in a few centres in the UK. This combined technique is the most pragmatic approach, when nuclear medicine facilities are limited. It does get over the problem of the few cases when the lymphatic channels are blocked by tumour and the sentinel nodes do not take up the tracer. Several series of this technique are now published, showing acceptable results, but there is no randomised study comparing this technique to a standard sentinel node biopsy.

Sentinel lymph node biopsy under local anaesthetic

A recent European study comprising 1018 patients who underwent sentinel lymph node biopsy under local anaesthetic has shown promising results.[24] Advantages of this technique include: (i) a reduction in operating time during breast surgery; (ii) no requirement for intra-operative pathological examination; and (iii) a positive impact on quality of life. Disadvantages included creating difficulties for further surgery due to sclerosis that makes future axillary dissection slow and difficult.[24]

Sentinel lymph node biopsy following neo-adjuvant chemotherapy

Small, single-institution studies have demonstrated that sentinel lymph node biopsy can be successfully performed after neo-adjuvant chemotherapy. Further prospective multicentre studies are needed to validate the false-negative rate of sentinel lymph node biopsy after neo-adjuvant chemotherapy.[25]

DUCTAL CARCINOMA *IN SITU*

Ductal carcinoma *in situ* is a proliferation of malignant epithelial cells within breast ducts without invasion of the basement membrane. The value of staging the axillary lymph nodes in ductal carcinoma *in situ* has been intensely controversial. By definition, ductal carcinoma *in situ* is pre-invasive and has no metastatic potential; therefore, a sentinel lymph node biopsy should not be necessary. Despite this, recent studies have shown that about 26% of women are diagnosed with an invasive lesion following excisional biopsy of ductal carcinoma *in situ*.[26] A sentinel lymph node biopsy should, therefore, be considered in patients who are at most risk of invasion. This group includes women with a palpable lesion, the presence of a mass using imaging or in patients undergoing mastectomy after a core or excisional biopsy diagnosis of ductal carcinoma *in situ*. Invasion may be missed in core biopsies due to sampling error and nodal metastases are found in about 1% of patients with ductal carcinoma *in situ* following axillary sampling. In summary, patients with ductal carcinoma *in situ* should be carefully selected to undergo the procedure of sentinel lymph node biopsy which carries a small risk of morbidity.

This procedure provides a useful adjunct in patients undergoing mastectomies and is not recommended in breast conserving surgery unless invasion is present.

Key point 6

- Sentinel lymph node biopsy is unnecessary in the management of pure ductal carcinoma *in situ* but is indicated if invasion is present.

AN OVERVIEW OF RECENT AXILLARY TRIALS

A summary of the recent major randomised trials undertaken is shown in Table 2.

Table 2 Randomised multicentre clinical trials of axillary surgery

TRIAL: IBCSG 23-01[27]	
Start date	2001
R of patients	Open *Total number* 1960
Arms	If SLN +ve for micrometastases, randomised to either (i) ALND or (ii) observation only
Goals	To determine the prognostic significance of microinvasion disease free survival, overall survival, quality of life and local recurrence. Primary endpoint is disease free survival
Follow-up	10 years
Results	Awaited
TRIAL: SNAC[28]	
Start date	2001
R of patients	Closed *Total number* 1088
Arms	Randomised to (i) SLNB alone +ALND if SLNB +ve. (ii) SLNB + ALND
Goals	The aim was to determine if SLNB (with ALND performed only if SLN +ve for metastases) results in less morbidity than ALND with equivalent cancer-related outcomes in early breast cancer.
Follow-up	10 years
Results	Early results have shown that women undergoing SLNB had fewer problems with arm swelling, movement and sensation problems with arm swelling.
TRIAL: ALMANAC[29]	
Start date	2000
R of patients	Closed Total number 1031
Arms	Randomised to: (i) ALND or sampling vs (ii) SLNB
Goals	To prove the clinical validity of SLNB and compare the 3 main outcome measures: (i) arm and axillary mobidity (ii) resource costs, (iii) quality of life. Secondary objective measured incidence of local recurrence
Follow-up	18 months
Results	Improved QOL and less arm morbidity in SLNB group. SLNB shown to accurately determine whether axillary metastases were present in patients with early stage breast cancer with clinically –ve axillary nodes. SLNB group had a reduced hospital stay.
TRIAL: ACOSOG Z0011[30] (closed prematurely due to slow accrual)	
Start date	1999
R of patients	Closed *Total number* 891 (target 1900)
Arms	Included clinically node –ve patients who had a +ve sentinel lymph node found at SLNB. Randomised to (i) completion ALND or (ii) no further surgery.
Goals	To assess whether overall survival for patients randomised to arm (ii) is equivalent to arm (i). To quantify and compare the surgical morbidities associated with SLNB plus ALND vs SLNB alone.
Follow-up	Lifelong
Results	Awaited

Table 2 *(cont'd)* Randomised controlled multicentre clinical trials of axillary surgery

TRIAL: NSABP-B32[31, 32]

Start date	1999
R of patients	Closed *Total number* 5611
Arms	Randomised to: (i) SLNB + immediate ALND or (ii) SLNB, only if SLNB +ve → ALND.
Goals	To determine if SLN resection could achieve the same therapeutic goals as conventional ALND but with decreased side-effects. Primary endpoints – morbidity, local recurrence rate, disease-free survival, overall survival.
Follow-up	Lifelong
Results	Survival, regional control and morbidity results awaited. Overall accuracy of SLNB was 97.1%. False –ve rate 9.8%[32] Differences in tumour location, type of biopsy, and number of SLNs removed significantly affected the false –ve rate.

TRIAL: IEO 185[33]

Start date	1998
R of patients	Closed *Total number* 516
Arms	Randomised to either (i) SLNB + ALND or (ii) SLNB. Those with a +ve SLNB immediately proceeded to a ALND in group (ii)., if the SLNB was –ve, no ALND was performed.
Goals	To determine the ability of SLNB vs ALND to discriminate between +ve and -ve axillae. Primary endpoint was to determine the staging power of SLNB as measured by the % of cases with axillary involvement compared with the % found in ALND
Follow-up	10 years
Results	Nodal positivity was similar in both groups demonstrating that SLNB alone can demonstrate axillary node metastases whilst reducing morbidity.

TRIAL: Chetty[22]

Start date	1987
R of patients	Closed *Total number* 466
Arms	Randomised to (i) ANC or (ii) ANS. Radiotherapy given to ANS arm if +ve lymph nodes.
Goals	To assess the extent of axillary dissection required, the need for radiotherapy to the axilla and the morbidity associated with these procedures.
Follow-up	4.1 years
Results	No difference was found in local, axillary or distant recurrence. No difference in 5 year overall survival. Morbidity was least in those who had ANS with no radiotherapy.

TRIAL: Forrest[23]

Start date	1980
R of patients	Closed *Total number* 417
Arms	After mastectomy, randomised to (i) ANC or (ii) ANS + radiotherapy if +ve lymph nodes.
Goals	To determine whether a standard 4 node axillary sample could accurately indicate the extent of local treatment required.
Follow-up	11 years
Results	No difference in survival, and little difference in locoregional relapse rates, between patients treated by node sampling or node clearance, even if +ve nodes are identified. ANC preferred where nodes +ve to ↓ morbidity of post sampling radiotherapy.

R of patients = recruitment of patients
ALND axillary lymph node dissection
SLNB sentinel lymph node biopsy
ANS axillary node sample
ANC axillary node clearance

TREATMENT OF THE INVOLVED AXILLA

Axillary lymph node dissection is mandatory if the nodes have been shown to harbour metastasis following pre-operative investigation or sentinel lymph node biopsy, the purpose being to improve overall survival. Adjuvant radiotherapy and or chemotherapy may be indicated depending on the size and grade of tumour and patient fitness.

AXILLARY NODE CLEARANCE

There is variation in the extent of axillary lymph node dissection between centres. An axillary clearance may refer to the removal of all lymphatic tissue in levels I, II and III, or simply levels I and II of the axilla. Patients should undergo this procedure if lymph nodes are positive or are likely to be positive. Where level I nodes are exclusively involved, clearing the axilla up to level II is acceptable. A level III clearance is preferred when nodes are heavily involved. The advantages of axillary lymph node dissection includes a lower local recurrence rate and avoidance of a second operation. It is, however, an unnecessary radical operation in patients who are node negative and is associated with reduced mobility of the shoulder and upper arm, lymphoedema, chronic pain, wound infection, seromas and nerve damage, and remains a major issue regarding reduced quality of life.

Key point 7

- Axillary lymph node dissection reduces the risk of axillary recurrence and avoids the need for a second operation.

SECOND AXILLARY SENTINEL NODE BIOPSIES FOR RECURRENT CANCERS

Approximately 5–10% of patients undergoing breast conserving surgery for breast cancer will develop tumour recurrence in the ipsilateral breast.[33] It was initially suggested that a primary sentinel lymph node biopsy would render a second procedure inaccurate due to the unpredictable patterns of lymphatic drainage in patients who had undergone previous surgery or radiotherapy. A recent study has, however, shown that a second sentinel lymph node biopsy after a previously negative sentinel lymph node biopsy can be performed in patients with ipsilateral breast cancer recurrence.[33]

CONCLUSIONS

- Current guidelines recommend sentinel lymph node biopsy as a surgical alternative to axillary lymph node dissection for patients with early breast cancer (T1 or T2) and clinically negative nodes. Patients with a negative sentinel lymph node biopsy do not require further treatment. However, if sentinel lymph node biopsy is positive, women should proceed with a completion axillary lymph node dissection. Sentinel lymph node biopsy is

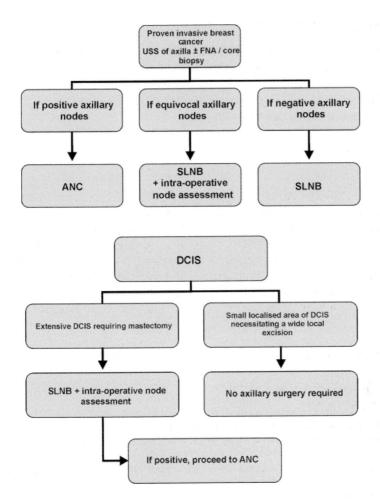

Fig. 5 Selection of patients for the various types of axillary surgery. USS, ultrasonography; DCIS, ductal carcinoma *in situ*; SLNB, sentinel lymph node biopsy; ANC, axillary node clearance; FNA, fine needle aspiration.

easy to learn and has a low rate of complications. Combining sentinel lymph node biopsy and axillary sampling may be preferable where there is limited access to a nuclear medicine department.

- Surgical staging of the axilla remains the gold standard because no reliable non-operative alternative has yet been demonstrated. Pre-operative sentinel lymph node biopsy may prove feasible; however, further research is required.

- Axillary lymph node dissection or radiotherapy continue to remain important in the treatment of women with involved nodes.

- Sentinel lymph node biopsy is not routinely recommended for patients diagnosed with pure ductal carcinoma *in situ*; however, it should be considered in women who are at high risk of harbouring occult invasive disease.

- The various recommendations for staging and treating patients with invasive breast cancer and ductal carcinoma *in situ* are summarised in Figure 5.

Key points for clinical practice

- Nodal involvement is considered to be the single most important prognostic indicator in women with breast cancer.

- In > 95% of breast cancers, cells metastasise to the axilla in a progressive manner from levels I to III.

- Clinical examination of the axilla is between 50–70% reliable in identifying metastatic lymph nodes.

- Removal of extra-axillary sentinel lymph nodes such as the internal mammary node is not routinely carried out.

- Injecting blue dye and radioactive tracer in the sub-areolar space in the segment of the tumour is an effective way of identifying the sentinel lymph node.

- Sentinel lymph node biopsy is unnecessary in the management of pure ductal carcinoma *in situ* but is indicated if invasion is present.

- Axillary lymph node dissection reduces the risk of axillary recurrence and avoids the need for a second operation.

References

1. Veronesi U. Value of limited surgery for breast cancer. *Semin Oncol* 1978; **5**: 395–402.
2. Hughes RJ, Jones C, Holland PA, Gateley CA. Prediction of axillary lymph node metastasis by size and grade of tumour – an aid for the discussion of axillary surgery in patients with operable disease. *Eur J Cancer Suppl* 2007; **5**: 21.
3. Veronesi U, Rilke F, Luini A *et al*. Distribution of axillary node metastases by level of invasion. *Cancer* 1987; **59**: 682–687.
4. Cody H. The sentinel node concept: a critique of the critique. *Breast* 2006; **15**: 571–574.
5. Benson JR, Querci della Rovere G. Management of the axilla in women with breast cancer. *Breast* 2007; **16**: 130–136.
6. Swinson C, Ravichandran D, Nayagam M *et al*. Preoperative axillary ultrasound and fine needle aspiration cytology of the axillary nodes in the diagnosis of axillary nodal involvement in breast cancer. San Antonio Breast Cancer Conference, December 2007.
7. Schwarz GF, Guiliano AE, Veronesi U. Proceedings of the Consensus Conference on the role of Sentinel Node Biopsy in Carcinoma of the Breast, April 19–22, 2001, Philadelphia, Pennsylvania. *Cancer* 2002; **94**: 2543–2551.
8. Goyal A, Newcombe R, Mansel R. Role of routine preoperative lymphoscintigraphy in sentinel node biopsy for breast cancer. On behalf of the ALMANAC Trialists Group. *Eur J Cancer* 2005; **41**: 238–243.
9. Goyal A, Newcombe GR, Mansel RE. Clinical relevance of multiple sentinel nodes in patients with breast cancer. *Br J Surg* 2005; **92**: 438–442.
10. Bauerfeind I, Galimberti V, Reitsamer R, Rutgers E, Untch M. Clinical aspects of sentinel lymph node biopsy. *Breast Care* 2007; **2**: 234–239.
11. Ozmen V, Neslihan C, Ozcinar B *et al*. Utility of internal mammary lymph node biopsy. 30th San Antonio Breast Cancer Conference, Abstract 3025, December 2007.
12. Golshan M, Martin WH, Dowlatshahi K. Sentinel lymph node biopsy lowers the rate of lymphoedema when compared with standard axillary lymph node dissection. *Am J Surg* 2003; **69**: 209–211.
13. Goyal A, Newcombe RG, Mansel R. Factors affecting failed localisation and false-negative rates of sentinel node biopsy in breast cancer – results of the ALMANAC

validation phase. Breast Cancer Research and Treatment, 2006.

14. Goyal A, Mansel RE, Douglas-Jones A, Woods V, Jasani B. Intra-operative assessment of sentinel lymph node using real time quantitative PCR versus delayed assessment of sentinel lymph node: a cost-effectiveness model. 30th San Antonio Breast Cancer Conference, Abstract 3012, December 2007.

15. Schem C, Maass N, Bauerschlag DO et al. One step nucleic acid amplification (OSNA) for intra-operative detection of lymph node metastases in breast cancer patients. 30th San Antonio Breast Conference, Abstract 3029, December 2007.

16. Purushotham AD, Ravichandran D, Lawrence D, Douglas-Jones A. Simultaneous dual isotope quantification of lymphatic flow to axillary nodes from intradermal and parenchymal tissue planes compared with nodal pathology in breast carcinoma; superiority of parenchymal injection for identification of the sentinel node. *Eur J Cancer* 2007; **5**: 20.

17. Ozmen V, Cabioglu N. Sentinel lymph node biopsy for breast cancer: current controversies. *Breast* 2006; **12**: S134–S142.

18. Ingram D, Hewett L, Maddern P. Anaphylaxis to patent blue during sentinel lymph node biopsy. *Aust NZ J Surg* 2004; **74**: 607–608.

19. Kawase K, Gayed IW, Hunt KK et al. Use of lymphoscintigraphy defines lymphatic drainage patterns before sentinel lymph node biopsy for breast cancer. *J Am Coll Surg* 2006; **203**: 64–72.

20. Barranger E, Uzan S, Kerrou K, Pitre S, Duval M, Charon Y. Place of a hand-held gamma camera (POCI) in the breast cancer sentinel lymph node. *Breast* 2007; **16**: 443–444.

21. Kissin M. Sentinel node biopsy for breast cancer: a ten year experience of >1000 cases from a single surgeon. *Eur J Cancer* 2007; **5**: 22.

22. Chetty U, Jack W, Prescott RJ, Tyler C, Rodger A. Management of the axilla in operable breast cancer treated by breast conservation: a randomized clinical trial. *Br J Surg* 2000;**87**:163-169.

23. Forrest APM, Everington D, McDonald CC, Steele RJC, Chetty U, Stewart HJ. The Edinburgh randomised trial of axillary sampling or clearance after mastectomy. *Br J Surg* 1995;**82**:1504-1508.

24. Luini A, Caldarella P, Gatti G et al. The sentinel node biopsy under local anaesthesia in breast cancer: advantages and problems, how the technique influenced the activity of a breast surgery department; update from the European Institute of Oncology with more than 1000 cases. *Breast* 2007; **16**: 527–532.

25. Classe JM et al. Sentinel lymph node biopsy after neoadjuvant chemotherapy for advanced breast cancer. Results of GANEA, a French prospective multicentric study. 30th San Antonio Breast Cancer Conference, Abstract 3004, December 2007.

26. Meijner P, Oldenburg HS, Loo CE, Niweg OG, Peterse JL, Rutgers EJ. Risk of invasion and axillary lymph node metastasis in ductal carcinoma in situ diagnosed by core-needle biopsy. *Br J Surg* 2007;94:952–956.

27. IBCSG 23-01 International Breast Cancer Study Group Trial of SLNB, USA.

28. Wetzig NR, Gratley GP, Owen U et al. SNAC Sentinel Node vs Axillary Clearance, Australia. Participation in the RAC Sentinel Node Biopsy Versus Axillary Clearance Trial. *ANZ J Surg* 2005; **75**: 98–100.

29. Mansel RE. ALMANAC Axillary Lymphatic Mapping Against Nodal Axillary Clearance Trial, UK. 27th San Antonio Breast Cancer Symposium, Abstract 18, 2004.

30. Lucci A. ACOSOG Z0011 American College Of Surgeons Oncology Group Z0011, USA. Surgical complications associated with sentinel lymph node dissection (SLND) plus axillary lymph node dissection, versus SLND alone in the American College of Surgeons Oncology Group (ACOSOG) Trial Z0011. *Ann Surg Oncol* 2006; 13: 4

31. Julian TB. NSABP-B32. National Surgical Adjuvant Breast & Bowel Project, USA. 27th San Antonio Breast Cancer Symposium, Abstract 12, 2004.

32. Krag D, Anderson SJ, Julian TB et al. for the National Surgical Adjuvant Breast and Bowel Project (NSABP). Technical outcomes of sentinel-lymph-node resection and conventional axillary-lymph-node dissection in patients with clinically node-negative breast cancer: results from the NSABP B-32 randomised phase III trial. *Lancet Oncol* 2007; **10**: 881–888.

33. IEO 185 European Institute of Oncology study 185. Mansel RE, Goyal A. European Studies on Breast Lymphatic Mapping. *Semin Oncol* 2004; **31**: 304–310.

Further Reading

34. Intra M, Trifiro G, Galimberti V, Gentilini O, Rotmensz N, Veronesi P. Second axillary sentinel node biopsy for ipsilateral breast tumour recurrence. *Br J Surg* 2007; **94**: 1216–1219.

35. Schüle J, Frisell J, Ingvar C, Bergkvist L. Sentinel node biopsy for breast cancer larger than 3 cm in diameter. *Br J Surg* 2007; **94**: 948–951.

36. Axelsson CK, Mouridsen HT, During M, Moller S. Axillary staging during surgery for breast cancer. *Br J Surg* 2007; **94**: 304–309.

37. Hussien M, Spence RAJ. Axillary lymph node clearance: overcoming the technical difficulties. *Breast* 2004; **13**: 133–138.

38. Gaston MS, Dixon JM. A survey of surgical management of the axilla in UK breast cancer patients. *Eur J Cancer* 2004; **40**: 1738–1742.

39. Popli MB, Sahoo M, Mehrotra N *et al*. Preoperative ultrasound-guided fine-needle aspiration cytology for axillary staging in breast carcinoma. *Australasian Radiol* 2006; **50**: 122–126.

40. Ung O, Tan M, Chua B, Barraclough B. Complete axillary dissection: a technique that still has relevance in contemporary management of breast cancer. *Aust NZ J Surg* 2006; **76**: 518–521.

41. Benson JR. Breast cancer and novel therapeutic treatments. *Eur Oncol Dis* 2007.

42. Van Deurzen CHM, Hobbelink MGC, Van Hillegersberg R, Van Diest PJ. Is there an indication for sentinel node biopsy in patients with ductal carcinoma *in situ* of the breast? A review. *Eur J Cancer* 2007; **43**: 993–1001.

43. Sprung J, Tully MJ, Ziser A. Anaphylactic reactions to isosulfan blue dye during sentinel node lymphadenectomy for breast cancer. *Anesth Analg* 2003; **96**: 1051–1053.

44. Komenaka IK, Bauer VP, Schnabel FR *et al*. Allergic reactions to isosulfan blue in sentinel lymph node mapping. *Breast J* 2005; **11**: 70–72.

45. Beenen E, de Roy van Zuidewijn DBW. Patients blue on patent blue: an adverse reaction during four sentinel node procedures. *Surg Oncol* 2005; **14**: 151–154.

46. MRI of the axilla will. *Breast Care* 2007; **5**: 273–348.

47. Veronesi U, Paganelli G, Viale G *et al*. Sentinel-lymph-node biopsy as a staging procedure in breast cancer: update of a randomised controlled study. *Lancet* 2006; **7**: 983–990.

48. Querci della Rovere G, Benson JR. A critique of the sentinel node concept. *Breast* 2006; **15**: 693–697.

49. Tanaka K, Yamamoto D, Kanematsu S, Okugawa H, Kamiyama Y. A four node axillary sampling trial on breast cancer patients. *Breast* 2006; 15: 203–209.

50. Langer I, Guller U, Berclaz G *et al*. Morbidity of sentinel lymph node biopsy (SLN) alone versus SLN and completion axillary lymph node dissection after breast cancer surgery. *Ann Surg* 2007; **245**: 3.

51. van Deurzen CHM, Hobbelink MGG, van Hillegersberg R, van Diest PJ. Is there an indication for sentinel node biopsy in patients with ductal carcinoma *in situ* of the breast? A review. *Eur J Cancer* 2007; **43**: 993–1001.

52. Argon A, Duygun U, Acar E *et al*. The use of periareolar intradermal Tc-99m tin colloid and peritumoural intraparenchymal isosulfan blue dye injections for determination of the sentinel lymph node. *Clin Nuclear Med* 2006; **31**: 795–800.

53. Husen M, Paaschburg B, Flyger H. Two-step axillary operation increases risk of arm morbidity in breast cancer patients. *Breast* 2006; **15**: 620–628.

54. Bleiweiss I. Sentinel lymph nodes in breast cancer after 10 years: rethinking basic principles. *Lancet* 2006; **7**: 686–692.

55. Tan M. Surmounting the challenges of sentinel lymph node biopsy for breast cancer in non-tertiary centres and community-based practices. *Aust NZ J Surg* 2006; **76**: 306–309.

56. Mansouri R, Chicken DW, Keshtgar MRS. Allergic reactions to patent blue dye. *J Surg Oncol* 20050

57. Mendez J, Fey J, Cody H, Borgen P, Sclafani LM. Can sentinel lymph node biopsy be omitted in patients with favourable breast cancer histology? *Ann Surg Oncol* 2005; **12**: 24–28.

Marcello Spampinato Hassan Elberm
Colin D. Johnson

14

Randomised clinical trials in surgery 2007

This chapter reviews all the randomised clinical trials (RCTs) dealing with general surgical questions, and published during 2007. We have also included some relevant systematic reviews and meta-analyses. The trials are grouped under sub-specialty headings for convenience, and each is summarised in a final Key Point. However, pressure of space has prevented detailed discussion, and the reader is urged to look at the original papers to appreciate fully the quality and implications of each.

In assessing RCTs, some measure of quality assessment is useful. We have applied the criteria of the Jadad score to highlight strengths and weaknesses. There are other systems for evaluation of trial quality; the reader should be aware of those features that make a trial report reliable and those which should encourage scepticism. The initials RCT do not in themselves imply valid conclusions.

LIVER SURGERY

DRAINS AND TUBES

After elective liver resections, drains are used for: (i) prevention of sub-phrenic or sub-hepatic fluid collection; (ii) identification and monitoring of postoperative bleeding; (iii) identification and drainage of any bile leak; and

Marcello Spampinato MD
Senior Clinical Fellow in HPB Surgery, University Department of Surgery, Southampton General Hospital, Southampton, UK

Hassan Elberm MRCS
Clinical Fellow in HPB Surgery, University Department of Surgery, Southampton General Hospital, Southampton, UK

Colin D. Johnson MChir FRCS (for correspondence)
Reader and Consultant Surgeon, University Surgical Unit, Southampton General Hospital, Tremona Road, Southampton SO16 6YD, UK. E-mail: c.d.johnson@soton.ac.uk

(iv) preventing the accumulation of ascites in cirrhotics. However, drains may increase the complication rates. In a recent systematic review,[1] five RCTs with 465 patients comparing drain versus no drain were included. Three of the five trials were of high methodological quality. There was no statistically significant difference between the two groups for any of the outcomes studied.

Many studies have questioned the use of a nasogastric tube in various surgical abdominal procedures[2] and its use has been recently associated with a higher incidence of pulmonary complications during abdominal surgery. In a randomised trial,[3] a total of 200 patients who had elective liver resection were randomised to have an nasogastric tube left in place after surgery until the passage of flatus or stool, or to have the nasogastric tube removed at the end of the operation. The primary objective of the study was to compare the incidence of postoperative complications. Overall surgical and medical morbidity rates were similar in the two groups, but the rate of pulmonary complications including pneumonia was significantly higher in the nasogastric tube group ($P = 0.047$). Secondary insertion of a nasogastric tube was required in 12% of patients in the no-tube arm, a mean ($\pm$ SD) of 3.9 ($\pm$ 1.9) days after surgery.

Key point 1

- Routine use of a drain or nasogastric tube after elective liver resection is unnecessary and may increase the rate of pulmonary complications.

LIMITING BLOOD LOSS DURING LIVER RESECTION

There is considerable controversy regarding whether or not vascular occlusion should be used to reduce blood loss during elective hepatectomies and which method is best to reduce blood loss. There is also considerable debate on the role of ischaemic preconditioning before vascular occlusion.

A recent systematic review[4] of 16 randomised trials has compared different types of vascular occlusion in terms of decreasing blood loss or decreasing ischaemia–reperfusion injury. Blood loss was significantly lower in vascular occlusion compared with no vascular occlusion. Plasma liver enzymes were significantly elevated in the vascular occlusion group compared with no vascular occlusion. There was no difference in mortality, liver failure, or other morbidities. Four of the five trials comparing resections done with or without vascular occlusion used intermittent vascular occlusion. There was no significant difference in the number of units transfused and patients needing transfusion. There was no difference in mortality, liver failure, or morbidity between total and selective methods of portal triad clamping with or without ischaemic preconditioning. However, ischaemic preconditioning was associated with lower blood loss and transfusion requirements.

Petrowsky *et al.*[5] compared ischaemic preconditioning of 10 min followed by continuous inflow clamping (maximum 75 min) versus intermittent inflow clamping (15/5 min cycles) in non-cirrhotic patients. The primary end-points were postoperative hepatocyte injury and blood loss during parenchyma transection.

To characterise the transaminase-based postoperative ischaemia–reperfusion injury, peak values as well as the area under the curve (AUC) of the postoperative course of AST and ALT were determined for the first 5 post-operative days. A total of 73 patients were randomised. The total blood loss and the blood loss during transection were significantly lower with ischaemic preconditioning. In 32% of patients with inflow clamping, parenchyma transection was interrupted due to significant bleeding during the 5-min reperfusion cycles, while this did not occur in the ischaemic preconditioning group ($P = 0.001$). These data are consistent with the systematic review.[4] Ischaemic preconditioning was associated with a significantly shorter transection time than inflow clamping, while the ischaemia time was comparable in both groups. There was no statistical difference between the two groups in term of ischaemia–reperfusion injury but, when this was assessed by age, it was found that ischaemic preconditioning protection becomes weaker with increasing age in a population older than 65 years; in contrast, the mean AUCAST remained unchanged in the different age populations of the inflow clamping group.

Key points 2 and 3

- There is no difference in terms of morbidity or mortality among the different type of inflow occlusion during liver resection in non-cirrhotic patients.

- Ischaemic preconditioning followed by continuous occlusion seems to be associated with a reduced blood loss during transection, but ischaemic preconditioning may not be

---

Glues are recommended as a means of improving peri-operative haemostasis and reducing biliary leakage after liver surgery. However, high-quality trials are few. In one such trial,[6] 300 patients undergoing hepatectomy were randomly assigned to fibrin glue application or control groups. There was an equal number of cirrhotic patients in the two arms. An absorbable collagen sponge was also applied with manual pressure, after spraying the glue. The primary end-point was to determine whether fibrin sealant could decrease postoperative bleeding and blood transfusion. There was no difference in postoperative drainage volume and characteristics of fluids between the two groups and transfusion requirements were the same. Two patients in both arms required a re-operation for postoperative bleeding. No significant difference was found in bile leak between the two groups. The authors' conclusion is that there are no advantages in using fibrin glue and application of a collagen, compared with a standard method of haemostasis. However, the use of the collagen sponge may have introduced a bias in the study. Moreover, the pre-operative coagulation status of the patients was not mentioned.

Reduction of central venous pressure has been employed successfully to reduce intra-operative blood loss during liver resection. A randomised controlled trial[7] has clarified the effectiveness of intra-operative blood salvage (normovolaemic haemodilution) in reducing central venous pressure and, therefore, blood loss. A total of 79 live liver donors were allocated intra-operatively to either blood salvage (blood volume equal to approximately 0.7% of the patient's body weight was collected before the liver transaction) or a control group. The primary outcome measure was blood loss during hepatic parenchymal division. Secondary outcome measures included central venous pressure at the start of the hepatic parenchymal division. The amount of blood loss during liver transection was significantly smaller in the blood salvage group than in the control group. The central venous pressure at the beginning of the liver parenchymal division was significantly lower in the blood salvage group than in the control group. The authors concluded that moderate intra-operative blood salvage safely and significantly reduced blood loss at the time of hepatic parenchymal division during liver graft procurement, although care must be exercised in expanding the indications of intra-operative blood salvage to other situations because the subjects of this trial were limited to those in good health and with normal liver function.

Key points 4 and 5

- The use of fibrin glue plus collagen sponge during elective liver resection is not justified.
- Intra-operative blood salvage effectively reduced the central venous pressure and bleeding during major liver resection for living donation. More studies are needed to expand the use of this method to resection for oncological purpose.

HEPATECTOMY FOR HEPATOCELLULAR CARCINOMA

The anterior approach technique has been advocated recently for large, right-liver tumours. However, there is no evidence to support its use routinely. In a recent prospective randomised controlled study,[8] 120 patients who had hepatocellular carcinoma larger than 5 cm in the right liver were assigned to an anterior-approach group or a conventional approach for right hepatectomy. Intra-operative blood loss of ≥ 2 litres occurred less frequently in the anterior approach group but there was no difference between the two groups in hospital mortality. However, all six deaths in the conventional-approach group were related to liver failure or multi-organ failure secondary to liver failure, whereas none occurred in the anterior-approach group. This is consistent with the suggestion that the anterior approach could contribute to better preservation of postoperative liver function by avoiding prolonged rotation and displacement of the hepatic lobes causing impairment of the afferent and efferent circulation of the remnant liver. The median overall cumulative survival of patients with stage II disease was ≥ 68.1 months in the anterior-approach group, which was significantly better than that of 23.7 months in the conventional-approach group. This difference was attributed to the availability of effective treatment of localised or solitary recurrences in 80% of patients with recurrent disease in the anterior-approach group. By contrast, effective treatment was only possible for 2 of 12 patients with recurrent disease in the conventional-approach group. The application of a no-touch technique during the anterior approach may have contributed to reduce the tumour vascular cell dissemination that may occur during the mobilisation of the liver.

The resection margin for cirrhotic Child–Pugh A patients undergoing liver resection for hepatocellular carcinoma remains controversial. In a randomised trial,[9] 169 patients with solitary hepatocellular carcinoma were stratified according to tumour size and randomised to undergo partial hepatectomy aiming grossly at a narrow (1 cm) or a wide resection margin (2 cm). The final resection margin was subsequently determined microscopically on the resected specimen and the results subjected to an intention-to-treat analysis. Randomisation was performed with stratification according to tumour size (≤ 2.0 cm, 2.1–5.0 cm, > 5 cm) although no mention of sample size according to stratification was reported. Primary and secondary end-points were overall survival and recurrence-free survival, respectively. The difference in the overall survival rates in the two groups was significant. However, when stratified according to tumour size, only patients with hepatocellular carcinoma ≤ 2 cm had a significant difference in overall survival rate between the two group. The overall 1-, 2-, 3- and 5-year recurrence-free survival rates reached a significant difference. However. when stratified according to tumour size, neither of the two group reached a statistically significant difference. A total of 75 (44.4%) patients in the study had developed recurrence but, interestingly, all 13 recurrences at the liver transection margin happened in the narrow-margin group while none occurred in the wide-margin group. The authors concluded that, for macroscopically solitary hepatocellular carcinoma, a 2-cm margin provided better survival outcome than a narrow resection margin aiming at 1 cm, especially for hepatocellular carcinoma ≤ 2 cm. Similar results have been reported in another randomised trial[10] with percutaneous radiofrequency ablation for hepatocellular carcinoma ≤ 2-cm diameter with the advantage of lower morbidity and mortality rates than liver resection.

Key points 6 and 7

- The anterior approach technique increases the overall survival rate in stage II disease and decreases blood loss during right hepatectomy performed for large hepatocellular carcinoma.

- A 2-cm margin provides a better survival rate in cirrhotic patients with hepatocellular carcinoma ≤ 2 cm undergoing liver resection. Radiofrequency ablation gives equivalent survival to liver resection for such patients.

PANCREATIC SURGERY

ANASTOMOTIC TECHNIQUE

There is continuing interest in technical adjustments to try to reduce leakage rates after pancreatic resection and anastomosis. Poon et al.[11] compared the results of pancreaticoduodenectomy with external drainage stent versus no stent for side-to-end pancreaticojejunostomy anastomosis in 120 patients. The stented group had a significantly lower rate of pancreatic fistula compared with the non-stented group (6.7% versus 20%, respectively).

Radiological or surgical intervention for pancreatic fistula was required in one patient of the stented group and four patients of the non-stented one, but there was no significant difference in overall morbidity and in-hospital mortality. Two patients (one in each group) died from pancreatic fistula. On accumulative analysis, pancreatic duct < 3 mm and no stenting were significant risks for pancreatic fistula.

By contrast, a group from Johns Hopkins reported a trial of internal pancreatic duct stenting following pancreaticoduodenectomy.[12] In the stent group, a 6-cm segment of a plastic paediatric feeding tube was used to stent the pancreaticojejunostomy anastomosis. The pancreatic fistula rate for the entire study population was 9.4%. The fistula rates with and without a stent with a hard pancreas were similar, at 1.7% and 4.8%, and with a soft pancreas were also similar, at 21.1% and 10.7%, respectively. The authors concluded that internal pancreatic duct stenting dose not decrease the frequency or the severity of postoperative pancreatic fistula.

Key point 8

- While there is a suggestion that external drainage of the pancreatic duct with a stent reduces the leakage rate of pancreaticojejunostomy after pancreaticoduodenectomy, internal pancreatic duct stenting does not decrease the frequency or the severity of postoperative pancreatic fistulas. Further trials may resolve this issue.

Peng et al.[42] compared leakage rate of a new binding technique with the conventional technique of pancreaticojejunostomy in 217 patients. Of the 111 patients randomised to the conventional group, pancreaticojejunostomy leakage occurred in 8 patients, while no patient in the 106 patients randomised to the binding group developed leakage ($P = 0.014$). Complications occurred in 41 patients (37%) in the conventional group compared with 26 patients (24.5%) in the binding group ($P = 0.048$). The mean postoperative hospital stay for the conventional group was 22.4 days (SD, 10.9 days), which was significantly longer than the binding group (18.4 days; SD, 4.7 days). The trial was not powered to detect differences in mortality rates.

Key point 9

- Binding pancreaticojejunostomy after pancreaticoduodenectomy significantly decreased postoperative complication and pancreaticojejunostomy leakage rates and shortened hospital stay when compared with conventional pancreaticojejunostomy.

PANCREATITIS

In patients with severe, necrotising pancreatitis, a number of studies have suggested that early, broad-spectrum antibiotics, often a carbapenem, might reduce the incidence of pancreatic and peripancreatic infections. Confirmation of benefit is lacking. Dellenger *et al.*[13] reported a multicentre, prospective, double-blind, placebo-controlled randomised study including 100 patients with necrotising pancreatitis allocated to meropenem (1 g i.v. every 8 h) or placebo starting within 5 days of the onset of symptoms for 7–21 days. The primary end-point was development of pancreatic or peripancreatic infection within 42 days following randomisation. Other end-points included: (i) time between onset of pancreatitis and the development of pancreatic or peripancreatic infection; (ii) all-cause mortality; (iii) requirement for surgical intervention; and (iv) development of non-pancreatic infections within 42 days following randomisation. Pancreatic or peripancreatic infections, surgical intervention and deaths occurred in similar numbers of patients in the two groups. This study is the largest to date in this patient group, and supports the growing view that antibiotics are unable to prevent infection of pancreatic necrosis.

Key point 10

- There is no support for early prophylactic antimicrobial use in patients with severe acute necrotising pancreatitis.

NUTRITION AND SYNBIOTICS AFTER PANCREATICODUODENECTOMY

Patients undergoing pancreatic resection carry several risk factors for bacterial infections. Recent data on overall bacterial infection rates in pancreatic surgery range between 20% and 30%.[14] Pre- and probiotics (synbiotics) are potentially useful for prevention of these infections.[15] In a single-centre RCT,[16] 80 patients undergoing pylorus preserving pancreaticoduodenectomy were randomised to receive either a combination of synbiotic enteral nutrition (two *Lactobacillus* spp., one *Pediococcus* spp., and one *Leuconostoc* spp. together with 4 fibres) or placebo (fibres only) starting the day before surgery and continuing for 8 days. All patients received enteral nutrition immediately postoperatively and a single-shot intravenous prophylaxis with cefuroxime and metronidazole 30 min before operaion. After that, antibiotics were only given in case of bacterial infection. The primary end-point was the occurrence of postoperative bacterial infection during the first 30 postoperative days. Infections occurred in 12.5% of the synbiotic group and 40% of the placebo group. There was no difference in ability to absorb the enteral nutrition in the two groups. The requirement for prolonged antibiotic therapy reached a statistically significant difference in favour of the synbiotic group.

Key point 11

- Enteral nutrition with synbiotics significantly reduces post-operative bacterial infections following pylorus preserving pancreaticoduodenectomy.

BILIARY SURGERY

Drains are often used after cholecystectomy to prevent abdominal collections. However, drain use may increase infective complications and delay discharge. In a recent systematic review,[17] six trials were analysed involving 741 patients randomised to drain versus no drain. Wound infection was significantly more likely in those with a drain (OR, 5.86; 95% CI, 1.05–32.70). Hospital stay was longer in the drain group and the number of patients discharged on the day of operation was significantly lower in the no-drain group (OR, 2.45; 95% CI, 0.00–0.57; one trial). The authors concluded that drain use after elective laparoscopic cholecystectomy increases wound infection rates and delays hospital discharge.

Key point 12

- There is no evidence to support the use of a drain after elective, uncomplicated, laparoscopic cholecystectomy.

UPPER GI SURGERY

REFLUX DISEASE

Two trials have shown the superiority of laparoscopic fundoplication over medical therapy for the long-term management of chronic reflux symptoms.

Anvari et al.[18] compared optimised medical therapy using a proton pump inhibitor ($n = 52$) with laparoscopic Nissen fundoplication ($n = 52$). Patients were monitored for 1 year. The primary end-point was frequency of gastro-oesophageal reflux disease symptoms. Surgical patients had improved symptoms, pH control, and overall quality-of-life health index after surgery at 1 year compared with the medical group. The overall gastro-oesophageal reflux disease symptom score at 1 year was unchanged in the medical patients, but improved in the surgical patients.

Mehta et al.[19] made similar observations in a longer follow-up. Between July 1997 and August 2001, 183 patients were randomised to either laparoscopic Nissen fundoplication or medical therapy for the treatment of reflux symptoms. After 12 months, those who had been randomised to medical therapy were offered the opportunity to have surgery: 54 of these patients had antireflux surgery, the remaining 38 did not. In October 2005, patients were followed up and asked to complete a reflux symptom questionnaire. In all three groups, there was a significant improvement in symptom score after the initial 12 months. However, those who later had surgery, despite having had optimal medical treatment beforehand, experienced further symptomatic improvement at long-term follow-up.

Key point 13

- Both optimal medical therapy and laparoscopic Nissen fundoplication are effective treatments for reflux disease. However, surgery offers additional benefit for those who have only partial symptomatic relief.

BARIATRIC SURGERY

Elsewhere in this volume, the subject of bariatric surgery is covered in some depth. One randomised trial[20] is considered here, reporting 5-year outcomes from a RCT in which 51 patients were randomly allocated to undergo either laparoscopic adjustable gastric banding (LAGB) using the pars flaccida technique or standard laparoscopic Roux-en-Y gastric bypass (LRYGB). Failure was considered a body mass index (BMI) of > 35 kg/m^2 at 5 years' postoperatively.

The mean operative time was 60 ± 20 min for the LAGB group and 220 ± 100 min for the LRYGB group ($P < 0.001$). One patient in the LAGB group was lost to follow-up. No patient died. Conversion to laparotomy was performed in 1 (4.2%) of 24 LRYGB patients because of a posterior leak of the gastrojejunal anastomosis. After 5 years, the LRYGB patients had significantly lower weight and BMI and a greater percentage of excess weight loss than did the LAGB patients. Weight loss failure (BMI > 35 kg/m^2 at 5 years) was observed in 9 (34.6%) of 26 LAGB patients and in 1 (4.2%) of 24 LRYGB patients ($P < 0.001$). Of the 26 patients in the LAGB group and 24 in the LRYGB group, 3 (11.5%) and 15 (62.5%) had a BMI of < 30 kg/m^2, respectively ($P < 0.001$).

Key point 14

- Standard laparoscopic Roux-en-Y gastric bypass results in better weight loss and a reduced number of failures compared with laparoscopic adjustable gastric banding, despite the significantly longer operative time and life-threatening complications.

GASTRIC CANCER

A multicentre, randomised, clinical trial was initiated by Kulig et al.[21] to evaluate the possible benefits of extended D2 (D2+; D2 plus removal of para-aortic nodes) lymphadenectomy after potentially curative resection of gastric cancer. Initial data on safety are presented. Of 781 patients screened, 275 were randomised to standard D2 ($n = 141$) or extended D2+ ($n = 134$) lymph-adenectomy. The overall morbidity rates were similar. Pre-existing cardiac disease, splenectomy, and excessive blood loss were identified as risk factors for overall and non-surgical complications. Postoperative mortality rates were 4.9% (95% CI, 1.4–8.5) and 2.2% (95% CI, 0–4.7), respectively.

Key point 15

- Interim safety analysis of D2 and extended D2 lymphadenectomy after potentially curative resection of gastric cancer did not show any significant difference in outcome between the two procedures.

ANTIBIOTIC PROPHYLAXIS IN GASTRIC CANCER SURGERY

The optimum duration of antimicrobial prophylaxis in elective gastric cancer surgery is still to be clarified. In a recent, multicentre, randomised, clinical trial,[22] 486 patients undergoing elective gastric surgery for cancer were randomised to receive either single- or multiple-dose antimicrobial prophylaxis regimens with cefazolin or ampicillin–sulbactam. The primary end-point was surgical-site infections. The overall incidence of surgical-site infections was 9.1% and no statistically significant difference was found between the two groups and the two types of antibiotic regimen used.

Key point

- A single dose of cefazolin or ampicillin–sulbactam is as effective as multiple doses for prevention of surgical-site infection during gastric cancer surgery.

TUBE FEEDING AFTER OESOPHAGECTOMY

Postoperative enteral feeding in patients undergoing major gastrointestinal surgery has been shown to reduce complications. However, the best delivery route has not been clarified. In a recent randomised trial,[23] 150 patients were randomised to receive either a jejunostomy or a nasoduodenal tube following oesophagectomy. The primary end-point was to assess the catheter-related complications. Of the patients in the jejunostomy group, 35% developed catheter-related complications compared to 30% in the nasoduodenal group ($P = 0.488$). The authors concluded that a nasoduodenal tube is an effective means of providing enteral feeding after oesophageal resection. However, these results should be interpreted with caution for the following reasons: (i) although the incidence of pneumonia was similar in both groups and could be related to the type of surgery, the nasoduodenal tube may have contributed to some of these cases and to the two cases of aspiration recorded in this group; and (ii) the rate of dislocation of the nasoduodenal tube was 23% but no information is given regarding the rate of re-insertion and associated complications.

COLORECTAL SURGERY

LAPAROSCOPIC CANCER SURGERY

Liang et al.[24] compared the oncological outcome between laparoscopic and open methods in the curative resection of stage 2 or 3 left-sided colon cancers, requiring take-down of the splenic flexure to facilitate curative left hemicolectomy. The primary end-point was time of tumour recurrence. The median follow-up was 40 months. The number of dissected lymph nodes was the same in each group, and the recurrence patterns were similar. The estimated cumulative recurrence rate for the surgery of stage 2 or 3 left-sided colon cancer was the same between laparoscopic and open methods.

Fleshman et al.[25] reported long-term outcome in a multi-institutional randomised trial including 872 patients, to compare laparoscopic-assisted or open colectomy. Patients were followed for 8 years, with 5-year data on 90% of patients. The primary end-point was time to recurrence, tested using a noninferiority trial design. Secondary end-points included overall survival and disease-free survival. Disease-free, 5-year survival (open, 68.4%; laparoscopic, 69.2%), overall 5-year survival (open, 74.6%; laparoscopic, 76.4%) and overall recurrence rates (open, 21.8%; laparoscopic, 19.4%) were similar in both groups. Sites of first recurrence were distributed similarly between the treatment arms (open – wound 0.5%, liver 5.8%, lung 4.6%, other 8.4%; laparoscopic – wound 0.9%, liver 5.5%, lung 4.6%, other 6.1%).

Jayne et al.[26] reported the long-term outcomes after laparoscopic-assisted surgery compared with conventional open surgery within the context of the UK MRC CLASICC trial: 794 patients were recruited (526 laparoscopic and 268 open). Overall, there were no differences in the long-term outcomes. Higher positivity of the circumferential resection margin was reported after laparoscopic anterior resection, but this did not translate into an increased incidence of local recurrence.

Key point 17

- Laparoscopic colectomy for curable colon cancer gives similar results to open surgery based on long-term oncological end-points in several prospective, randomised trials.

COLON POUCH

Fazio et al.[27] reported a long-term, randomised, controlled trial to compare functional outcomes and quality of life (QoL) after coloplasty, colonic J-pouch, or a straight anastomosis in the treatment of low rectal cancer. Patients with low rectal cancer were randomised intra-operatively to coloplasty (CP-1) or straight anastomosis if J-pouch was not feasible, or J-pouch or coloplasty (CP-2) if a J-pouch was feasible. Patients were followed for 24 months with SF-36 surveys to evaluate QoL. Bowel function was measured quantitatively and using Fecal Incontinence Severity Index (FISI). Urinary function and sexual function were also assessed. All 364 randomised patients were evaluated for complications and recurrence. No significant difference was observed in complications among the four groups. Functional outcome was assessed in 297 patients at 24 months. There was no difference in bowel function between the CP-1 and straight anastomosis groups. J-pouch patients had fewer bowel movements, less clustering, used fewer pads and had a lower FISI than the CP-2 group. Other parameters were not statistically different. QoL scores at 24 months were similar for each of the four groups.

Key point 18

- In patients undergoing a restorative resection for low rectal cancer, a colonic J-pouch offers significant advantages in function over a straight anastomosis or a coloplasty. In patients who cannot have a pouch, coloplasty and straight anastomosis give similar functional results.

Recent studies have suggested that mechanical bowel preparation does not lower the risk of postoperative septic complications after elective colorectal surgery. Jung *et al.*[28] addressed this question in elective colonic surgery. A total of 1505 patients were randomised to mechanical bowel preparation or no mechanical bowel preparation before open elective surgery for cancer, adenoma or diverticular disease of the colon. Primary end-points were cardiovascular, general infections and surgical-site complications within 30 days, and secondary end-points were death and re-operations within 30 days. A total of 1343 patients were evaluated, 686 randomised to mechanical bowel preparation and 657 to no mechanical bowel preparation. There were no significant differences in overall complications between the two groups: cardiovascular complications occurred in 5·1% and 4·6%, respectively, general infectious complications in 7·9% and 6·8% and surgical-site complications in 15·1% and 16·1%. At least one complication was recorded in 24·5% of patients who had mechanical bowel preparation and 23·7% who did not.

Key point 19

- Mechanical bowel preparation does not lower the complication rate and can be omitted before elective colonic resection.

The use of prophylactic antibiotics in elective colorectal surgery is essential. Although single-dose prophylactic antibiotics are recommended, the efficacy of single-dose cephalosporin without metronidazole and oral antibiotics is not fully proven. Fujita *et al.*[29] carried out a multicentre, randomised trial of single dose versus three doses of the second-generation cephalosporin, cefmetazole. Patients were randomised to either a single dose of cefmetazole just before skin incision or a 3-dose group given two additional doses of cefmetazole every 8 h. The main outcome measures were incidences of incisional surgical-site infection, organ or space surgical-site infection, and all other infectious complications within 30 days after surgery. A total of 384 patients were enrolled. Seven patients were excluded because of additional surgery or the inability to tolerate mechanical preparation. The incidence of incisional surgical-site infection was higher in the single-dose group (27 of 190; 14.2%) than in the 3-dose group (8 of 187; 4.3%). Incidences of organ or space surgical-site infection and other postoperative infectious diseases did not differ significantly between the two groups. In multivariate analysis, antibiotic dose was the only significant factor related to the incidence of incisional surgical-site infection.

Key point 20

- Three-dose cefmetazole administration is significantly more effective for prevention of incisional surgical-site infection than single-dose antibiotic administration.

SENTINEL LYMPH NODE BIOPSY

The principal role of sentinel lymph node sampling and ultrastaging in colon cancer is enhanced staging accuracy. The utility of this technique for patients with colon cancer remains controversial. A multicentre, randomised trial[30] was conducted to determine if focused assessment of the sentinel lymph node with step sectioning and immunohistochemistry enhances the ability to stage the regional nodal basin over conventional histopathology in patients with resectable colon cancer. Between August 2002 and April 2006, 161 patients with stage I–III colon cancer were randomly assigned to standard histopathological evaluation or sentinel lymph node mapping (*ex vivo*, subserosal, peritumoural, 1% isosulfan blue dye) and ultrastaging with pan-cytokeratin immuno-histochemistry in conjunction with standard histopathology. Sentinel lymph node-positive disease was defined as individual tumour cells or cell aggregates identified by haematoxylin and eosin (H&E) and/or immuno-histochemistry. Primary end-point was the rate of nodal up-staging. Significant nodal up-staging was identified with sentinel lymph node ultrastaging (control 38.7% versus sentinel lymph node 57.3%; $P = 0.019$). When sentinel lymph nodes with cell aggregates ≤ 0.2 mm in size were excluded, no statistically significant difference in node-positive rate was apparent between the control and sentinel lymph node arms (38.7% versus 39.0%; $P = 0.97$). However, a 10.7% (6 of 56) nodal up-staging was identified by evaluation of H&E-stained step sections of sentinel lymph nodes among study arm patients who would have otherwise been staged node-negative by conventional pathological assessment alone.

Key point 21

- Sentinel lymph node mapping, step sectioning, and immuno-histochemistry identifies small-volume nodal disease and improves staging in patients with resectable colon cancer. The clinical significance of colon cancer micrometastasis in sentinel lymph nodes remains unclear.

VASCULAR SURGERY

ROUTINE OR OPTIONAL STENTING?

Previous data showed good early results with primary stenting with self-expanding nitinol stents of the superficial femoral artery compared with balloon angioplasty with optional stenting. Schillinger *et al.*[31] now report 2-year data on re-stenosis and clinical outcomes of these patients. Of 104 patients with chronic limb ischaemia and superficial femoral artery obstructions, 98 (94%) could be followed up until 2 years after intervention. Re-stenosis rates were 46% (21 of 46) versus 69% (36 of 52) in favour of primary stenting compared with balloon angioplasty with optional secondary stenting by an intention-to-treat analysis. Patients in the primary stent group showed a trend toward better treadmill walking capacity (average 302 m versus 196 m; $P = 0.12$)

and better ankle brachial index values (average 0.88 versus 0.78; $P = 0.09$) at 2 years. Re-intervention rates tended to be lower after primary stenting (17 of 46 [37.0%] versus 28 of 52 [53.8%]; $P = 0.14$). The authors concluded that primary stenting with self-expanding nitinol stents for the treatment of superficial femoral artery obstructions yields a sustained morphological benefit and a non-significant trend toward clinical benefit compared with balloon angioplasty with optional stenting.

Key point 22

• Primary stenting with self-expanding nitinol stents of the superficial femoral artery is no better than balloon angioplasty with optional stenting and new data do not justify a change from current practice.

MEDICAL TREATMENT IN PERIPHERAL VASCULAR DISEASE

Two large studies have examined the benefits of medical therapy aimed at reduction of disease progression and cardiovascular mortality in patients with peripheral vascular disease.

The first trial[32] assessed the prophylactic efficacy of aspirin and a high-dose antioxidant vitamin combination to reduce the risk of a first vascular event (myocardial infarction, stroke, vascular death) and critical limb ischaemia. A total of 366 out-patients with stage I–II disease were entered into one of four treatment groups: (i) oral aspirin (100 mg daily); (ii) oral antioxidant vitamins (600 mg vitamin E, 250 mg vitamin C and 20 mg β-carotene daily); (iii) both; or (iv) neither, given for 2 years. Complete follow-up was achieved in 210 patients. Seven of 185 patients allocated aspirin and 20 of 181 allocated placebo suffered a major vascular event (risk reduction 64%; $P = 0.022$); five and eight patients, respectively, suffered critical leg ischaemia (total 12 versus 28; $P = 0.014$). There was no evidence that antioxidant vitamins were beneficial (16 of 185 versus 11 of 181 vascular events). Neither treatment was associated with any significant increase in adverse events. These findings suggest that low-dose aspirin reduces the incidence of vascular events by 26%.

In the second trial,[33] the investigators assigned patients with peripheral arterial disease to combination therapy with an antiplatelet agent and an oral anticoagulant agent (target international normalised ratio [INR], 2.0–3.0) or to antiplatelet therapy alone to assess effect on vascular events. A total of 2161 patients were followed for a mean of 35 months. Myocardial infarction, stroke, severe ischaemia, or death from cardiovascular causes occurred in 172 (15.9%) of 1080 patients receiving combination therapy as compared with 188 (17.4%) of 1081 patients receiving antiplatelet therapy alone. Life-threatening bleeding occurred in 43 patients receiving combination therapy (4.0%) as compared with 13 patients receiving antiplatelet therapy alone (1.2%; relative risk, 3.41; 95% CI, 1.84–6.35; $P < 0.001$). These data demonstrate that, in patients with peripheral arterial disease, the combination of an oral anticoagulant and antiplatelet therapy was not more effective than antiplatelet therapy alone in preventing major cardiovascular complications and was associated with an increase in life-threatening bleeding.

EXERCISE AFTER BYPASS

A study has evaluated the efficacy of an exercise programme after peripheral arterial bypass surgery.[34] Patients undergoing bypass surgery were randomised to standard pre-operative and postoperative care, or to a supervised exercise programme of twice-weekly treadmill assessments from 4–10 weeks' postoperatively. Ankle-brachial pressure indices and haemodynamic measurements were recorded before and after exercise. The mean increase of maximum walking distance was 3.8% in group I and 175.4% in group II. There was a significant difference between the groups in the mean ankle-brachial pressure indices increase at the second assessment (0.08 versus 0.23). The authors concluded that a supervised exercise programme leads to greater improvement after lower limb bypass surgery for ischaemia, but the feasibility of a formal exercise programme would be limited by the reluctance of patients to participate, both in the short-term and long-term.

EARLY TREATMENT OF CLAUDICATION

Timing of the first intervention in claudication is controversial. A single-centre, prospective, randomised trial[35] compared optimal medical treatment (OMT) only with OMT combined with percutaneous transluminal angioplasty (OMT+PTA) in patients with intermittent claudication. Quality of life (QoL) was the primary outcome measure. Only 56 patients with disabling intermittent claudication fulfilled the stringent inclusion criteria. After 2 years of follow-up, some variables from the QoL assessment showed a significant improvement in favour of the OMT+PTA group. Ankle pressures, the treadmill walking distances and the VAS were significantly improved in the group treated with OMT+PTA, compared to the group treated with OMT.

BREAST SURGERY

In a single blind RCT, Rodd et al.[36] compared the outcome of patients undergoing simple mastectomy using either the standard scalpel blade technique or the bipolar cutting scissor technique. Each arm of the trial contained 30 patients. The two primary outcome measures were intra-operative blood loss and the operating time. These were significantly less in the scissors group which also had better chest wall clearance and skin flap development as assessments of surgical completeness of mastectomy.

Key point 25

- The use of electric scissors reduces the intra-operative blood loss and operating time during mastectomy.

Rodier et al.[37] attempted to determine the optimal injection path for blue dye and radiocolloid for sentinel lymph node biopsy in early breast cancer. They compared the peritumoural injection site to the peri-areolar site in 449 patients. The detection rate of axillary sentinel lymph node by lymphoscintigraphy was significantly higher in the peri-areolar group (85.2%) than in the peritumoural group (73.2%). Intra-operative detection rate by blue dye and/or gamma probe was similar (99.11%) in both groups. The rate of sentinel lymph node detection was similar in the two groups: 95.6% versus 93.8% with blue dye and 98.2% versus 96.0% by the probe, respectively. The number of sentinel lymph nodes detected by lymphoscintigraphy and by probe was significantly higher in the peri-areolar group than in the peritumoural group (mean 1.5 versus 1.2 and 1.9 versus 1.7). The blue and hot concordance was 95,6% in the peri-areolar group and 91.5% in the peritumoural group. The mean *ex vivo* count of the sentinel lymph node was significantly higher in the peri-areolar group than the peritumoural group ($P < .0001$).

Key point 26

- In sentinel lymph node biopsy in early breast cancer, peri-areolar injection has a high detection rate and high concordance between blue dye and the radiotracer and is, therefore, superior to peritumoural injection.

EMERGENCY SURGERY

Morino et al.[38] reported a prospective, randomised, single-institution trial to assess the role of early laparoscopy in the management of non-specific abdominal pain in young women. Women aged 13–45 years, admitted as an emergency with non-specific abdominal pain, were included. Exclusion criteria were pregnancy, previous appendicectomy, contra-indications to laparoscopy, diagnosis of malignancy, or chronic disease. Non-specific abdominal pain was defined as abdominal pain in the right iliac or hypogastric area lasting more than 6 h and less than 8 days, without fever, leukocytosis, or obvious peritoneal signs, and uncertain diagnosis after physical examination and baseline investigations including abdominal ultrasonography. Patients were randomly assigned to early (< 12 h from admission) laparoscopy ($n = 53$) or to clinical observation ($n = 51$). A diagnosis was established in hospital in 83% of the laparoscopy group and in 45% of the clinical observation group. Twenty clinical-observation patients (39%) were operated during observation because of worsening of symptoms or appearance of peritoneal signs. Mean length of hospital stay was 3.7 ± 0.4 days in the laparoscopy and 4.7 ± 2.4 days in the clinical observation groups; no differences were found regarding mortality, morbidity, radiation dose, and analgesia. Abdominal pain was present at 3 months and 12 months from discharge in 20% and 16% of patients in the laparoscopy group and in 52% and 25% in the clinical observation group. Six patients in the clinical observation group required re-admission for surgery.

Key point 27

- Compared with active clinical observation, early laparoscopy did not show a clear benefit in women with non-specific abdominal pain. A higher number of diagnoses and a shorter hospital stay in the laparoscopy group did not lead to a significant reduction in symptom recurrences at 1 year.

POSTOPERATIVE MANAGEMENT

EARLY ENTERAL NUTRITION

Restriction of oral intake, and routine use of a nasogastric tube may be unnecessary in elective abdominal surgery. In a randomised trial,[39] 128 patients were allocated to receive a conventional postoperative dietary regimen or a free diet of their own choice after open colorectal and vascular surgery. The primary end-point was re-insertion of an nasogastric tube. Secondary outcome measures were interval between operation and tolerance of a normal diet, duration of hospital stay and complications. There was no difference in the two groups in the need for re-insertion of a nasogastric tube, time to normal bowel sounds, time to passage of flatus, time to first defecation, and hospital stay. Patients in the free-diet group, however, tolerated a meal containing solid food earlier than those in the conventional group. The authors' conclusion was that most patients tolerate early resumption of oral intake after operation, despite incomplete recovery of gastrointestinal function, and this does not lead to a higher postoperative complication rate. However these results should be interpreted with caution. In fact, there was no effort to standardise the primary outcome and to blind the study by leaving to the responsible physician the decision to re-insert the nasogastric tube and evaluate the bowel function.

> ## Key point 28
>
> - Early enteral nutrition may speed recovery from elective abdominal surgery.

PAIN RELIEF AFTER ABDOMINAL SURGERY

Typically, postoperative pain control is established and maintained using epidural and/or intravenous opioids for the first 24–48 h after surgery, with a transition to oral opioids thereafter. In a recent double-blind randomised trial,[40] 331 patients undergoing abdominal surgery with an incision ≥ 5 cm and experiencing moderate-to-severe pain within 30 h from surgery and expected to require oral narcotics therapy for ≥ 48 h were randomised to receive Oxymorphone immediate release 10 mg or 20 mg, Oxycodone immediate release 15 mg (used as active control group), or placebo every 4–6 h after the previous dose for 48 h. The primary end-point was the median time to study medication discontinuation for all causes which was significantly longer for all active treatments compared with placebo. Oxymorphone immediate release 20 mg was significantly more effective than placebo over the 6-h single-dose evaluation. With multiple dosing, all active treatment groups had significantly reduced pain intensities compared with placebo.

> ## Key point 29
>
> - Oxymorphone immediate release given every 4–6 h for up to 48 h provided good analgesia for moderate-to-severe pain in adult patients undergoing open abdominal surgery.

PERI-OPERATIVE SYSTEMIC WARMING

Intra-operative systemic warming has been shown to improve outcomes of surgery. Pre-operative warming has not been investigated. In a recent randomised trial,[41] 103 patients undergoing mostly open colorectal surgery were randomised to receive pre-operative warming for 2 h before surgery using a conductive carbon polymer mattress or standard treatment. Both groups were warmed during the operation. Primary end-point was the number of postoperative complications. Significantly fewer patients in the warming group (32%) developed any complications than in the control group (54%). Moreover, patients in the warming group had significantly less blood loss (median, 200 ml) than the control group (median, 400 ml). However, these results should be interpreted with caution because the inclusion criteria specified only well-nourished patients.

> ## Key point 30
>
> - Pre-operative warming may reduce postoperative complication rates.

References

1. Gurusamy KS, Samraj K, Davidson BR. Routine abdominal drainage for uncomplicated liver resection. Cochrane Database Syst Rev 2007; CD006232.

2. Nelson R, Edwards S, Tse B. Prophylactic nasogastric decompression after abdominal surgery. Cochrane Database Syst Rev 2007; CD004929.

3. Pessaux P, Regimbeau JM, Dondero F et al. Randomized clinical trial evaluating the need for routine nasogastric decompression after elective hepatic resection. Br J Surg 2007; **94**: 297–303.

4. Gurusamy KS, Kumar Y, Sharma D et al. Methods of vascular occlusion for elective liver resections. Cochrane Database Syst Rev 2007; CD006409.

5. Petrowsky H, McCormack L, Trujillo M et al. A prospective, randomized, controlled trial comparing intermittent portal triad clamping versus ischemic preconditioning with continuous clamping for major liver resection. Ann Surg 2006; **244**: 921–928.

6. Figueras J, Llado L, Miro M et al. Application of fibrin glue sealant after hepatectomy does not seem justified: results of a randomized study in 300 patients. Ann Surg 2007; **245**: 536–542.

7. Hashimoto T, Kokudo N, Orii R et al. Intraoperative blood salvage during liver resection: a randomized controlled trial. Ann Surg 2007; **245**: 686–691.

8. Liu CL, Fan ST, Cheung ST et al. Anterior approach versus conventional approach right hepatic resection for large hepatocellular carcinoma: a prospective randomized controlled study. Ann Surg 2006; **244**: 194–203.

9. Shi M, Guo RP, Lin XJ et al. Partial hepatectomy with wide versus narrow resection margin for solitary hepatocellular carcinoma: a prospective randomized trial. Ann Surg 2007; **245**: 36–43.

10. Chen MS, Li JQ, Zheng Y et al. A prospective randomized trial comparing percutaneous local ablative therapy and partial hepatectomy for small hepatocellular carcinoma. Ann Surg 2006; **243**: 321–328.

11. Poon RTP, Fan ST, Lo CM et al. External drainage of the pancreatic duct with a stent to reduce leakage rate of pancreaticojejunostomy after pancreaticoduodenectomy. Ann Surg 2007; **246**: 425–435.

12. Winter JM, Cameron JL, Campbell KA et al. Does pancreatic duct stenting decrease the rate of pancreatic fistula following pancreaticoduodenectomy? Results of a prospective randomized trial. J Gastroenterol 2006; **10**: 1280–1290.

13. Dellinger EP, Tellado JM, Soto NE et al. Early antibiotic treatment for severe acute necrotizing pancreatitis. Ann Surg 2007; **245**: 674–683.

14. Di Carlo V, Gianotti L, Balzano G et al. Complications of pancreatic surgery and the role of perioperative nutrition. Dig Surg 1999; **16**: 320–326.

15. Rayes N, Hansen S, Seehofer D et al. Early enteral supply of fiber and Lactobacilli versus conventional nutrition: a controlled trial in patients with major abdominal surgery. Nutrition 2002; **18**: 609–615.

16. Rayes N, Seehofer D, Theruvath T et al. Effect of enteral nutrition and synbiotics on bacterial infection rates after pylorus-preserving pancreatoduodenectomy: a randomized, double-blind trial. Ann Surg 2007; **246**: 36–41.

17. Gurusamy KS, Samraj K, Mullerat P et al. Routine abdominal drainage for uncomplicated laparoscopic cholecystectomy. Cochrane Database Syst Rev 2007; CD006004.

18. Anvari M, Allen C, Marshall J et al. A randomized controlled trial of laparoscopic Nissen fundoplication versus proton pump inhibitors for treatment of patients with chronic gastroesophageal reflux disease: one-year follow-up. Surg Innovat 2006; **13**: 238–249.

19. Mehta S, Bennett J, Mahon D, Rhodes M. Prospective trial of laparoscopic Nissen fundoplication versus proton pump inhibitor therapy for gastroesophageal reflux disease: seven-year follow-up. J Gastrointest Surg 2006; **10**: 1312–1317.

20. Angrisani L, Lorenzo M, Borrelli V. Laparoscopic adjustable gastric banding versus Roux-en-Y gastric bypass: 5-year results of a prospective randomized trial. Surg Obesity Rel Dis 2007; **3**: 127–133.

21. Kulig J, Popiela T, Kolodziejczyk P, Sierzega M, Szczepanik A, on behalf of the Polish Gastric Cancer Study Group. Standard D2 versus extended D2 (D2+) lymphadenectomy for gastric cancer: an interim safety analysis of a multicenter, randomized, clinical trial. Am J Surg 2007; **193**: 10–15.

22. Mohri Y, Tonouchi H, Kobayashi M *et al*. Randomized clinical trial of single- versus multiple-dose antimicrobial prophylaxis in gastric cancer surgery. *Br J Surg* 2007; **94**: 683–688.

23. Han-Geurts IJ, Hop WC, Verhoef C *et al*. Randomized clinical trial comparing feeding jejunostomy with nasoduodenal tube placement in patients undergoing oesophagectomy. *Br J Surg* 2007; **94**: 31–35.

24. Liang JT, Huang KC, Lai HS, Lee PH, Jeng YM. Oncological results of laparoscopic versus open surgery for stage 2 and 3 left-sided colon cancers. *Ann Surg Oncol* 2007; **14**: 109–117.

25. Fleshman J, Sargent DJ, Green E *et al*., for The Clinical Outcomes of Surgical Therapy Study Group. Laparoscopic colectomy for cancer is not inferior to open surgery based on 5-year data from the COST Study Group Trial. *Ann Surg* 2007; **246**: 655–664.

26. Jayne DG, Guillou PJ, Thorpe H *et al*. Randomized clinical trial of laparoscopic-assisted resection of colorectal carcinoma: 3-year results of the UK MRC CLASICC Trial Group. *J Clin Oncol* 2007; **25**: 3061–3068.

27. Fazio VW, Zutshi M, Remzi FH *et al*. A randomized multicenter trial to compare long-term functional outcome, quality of life, and complications of surgical procedures for low rectal cancers. *Ann Surg* 2007; **246**: 481–490.

28. Jung B, Pahlman L, Nystrom PO, Nisson E for the Mechanical Bowel Preparation Study Group. Multicentre randomized clinical trial of mechanical bowel preparation in elective colonic resection. *Br J Surg* 2007; **94**: 689–695.

29. Fujita S, Saito N, Yamada T *et al*. Randomized, multicenter trial of antibiotic prophylaxis in elective colorectal surgery. Single dose vs 3 doses of a second-generation cephalosporin without metronidazole and oral antibiotics. *Arch Surg* 2007; **142**: 657–661.

30. Stojadinovic A, Nissan A, Protic M *et al*. Prospective randomized study comparing sentinel lymph node evaluation with standard pathologic evaluation for the staging of colon carcinoma. Results from the United States Military Cancer Institute Clinical Trials Group Study G1-0l. *Ann Surg* 2007; **245**: 846–857.

31. Schillinger M, Sabeti S, Dick P *et al*. Sustained benefit at 2 years of primary femoropopliteal stenting compared with balloon angioplasty with optional stenting. *Circulation* 2007; **115**: 2745–2749.

32. Critical Leg Ischaemia Prevention Study (CLIPS) Group, Catalano M, Born G, Peto R. Prevention of serious vascular events by aspirin amongst patients with peripheral arterial disease: randomized, double-blind trial. *J Intern Med* 2007; **261**: 276–284.

33. Warfarin Antiplatelet Vascular Evaluation Trial Investigators, Anand S, Yusuf S, Xie C, Pogue J *et al*. Oral anticoagulant and antiplatelet therapy and peripheral arterial disease. *N Engl J Med* 2007; **357**: 217–227.

34. Badger SA, Soong CV, O'Donnell ME, Boreham CA, McGuigan KE. Benefits of a supervised exercise program after lower limb bypass surgery. *Vasc Endovasc Surg* 2007; **41**: 27–32.

35. Nylaende M, Abdelnoor M, Stranden E *et al*. The Oslo balloon angioplasty versus conservative treatment study (OBACT) – the 2-years results of a single centre, prospective, randomised study in patients with intermittent claudication. *Eur J Vasc Endovasc Surg* 2007; **33**: 3–12.

36. Rodd CD, Vamsi R, Holly-Archer F, Clark A. Pereira JH. Randomized clinical trial comparing two mastectomy techniques. *World J Surg* 2007; **31**: 1164–1168.

37. Rodier JF, Velten M, Wilt M *et al*. Prospective multicentric randomized study comparing periareolar and peritumoral injection of radiotracer and blue dye for the detection of sentinel lymph node in breast sparing procedures: FRANSENODE Trial. *J Clin Oncol* 2007; **25**: 3664–3669.

38. Morino M, Pellegrino, L, Castagna E, Farinella E, Mao P. Acute nonspecific abdominal pain. A randomized controlled trial comparing early laparoscopy versus clinical observation. *Ann Surg* 2006; **244**: 881–888.

39. Han-Geurts IJ, Hop WC, Kok NF *et al*. Randomized clinical trial of the impact of early enteral feeding on postoperative ileus and recovery. *Br J Surg* 2007; **94**: 555–561.

40. Aqua K, Gimbel JS, Singla N *et al*. Efficacy and tolerability of Oxymorphone immediate release for acute postoperative pain after abdominal surgery: a randomized, double-blind, active- and placebo-controlled, parallel-group trial. *Clin Ther* 2007; **29**: 1000–1012.

41. Wong PF, Kumar S, Bohra A *et al*. Randomized clinical trial of perioperative systemic warming in major elective abdominal surgery. *Br J Surg* 2007; **94**: 421–426.

42. Peng SY, Wang JW, Lau WY *et al*. Conventional versus binding pancreaticojejunostomy after pancreaticoduodenectomy. A prospective randomized trial. *Ann Surg* 2007; **245**: 692–698.

Index

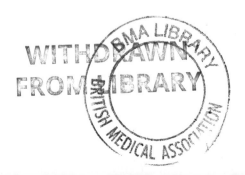